The New

E FOR ADDITIVES

THE COMPLETELY REVISED
BESTSELLING E NUMBER GUIDE

Maurice Hanssen
with Jill Marsden
B.Sc., Dip.Ecol., Dip.Ed.

THORSONS PUBLISHING GROUP
Wellingborough, Northamptonshire
Rochester, Vermont

First published September 1987

British Library Cataloguing in Publication Data

Hanssen, Maurice
The new E for additives: the completely
revised bestselling E number guide.
1. Food additives — Tables
I. Title   II. Marsden, Jill   III. Hanssen,
Maurice. E for additives
664'.06'0212   TX553.A3

ISBN 0-7225-1562-6

Printed and bound in Great Britain

1 3 5 7 9 10 8 6 4 2

The New E FOR ADDITIVES

The best consumer guide in Europe on additives
in food, providing you with all the facts to make
informed decisions about what you buy.

Contents

Foreword by Lord Ennals   7
Foreword to First Edition by Leslie Kenton   9
Introduction   10
1. How to Read the Label   13
2. Why Are There Still Secret Ingredients?   27
3. Golden Eggs and Pink-Fleshed Fish   35
4. The Colour Problem   38
5. Flavourings   43
6. P for Pesticides?   45
7. Is It Kosher?   47
8. Do Additives Affect Ability?   49
9. Hyperactivity in Children   53
10. The Avoidable 57 Additives   57
11. The Natural Opportunity for Profit   61
12. The E Number Categories   63
Appendix I An Introduction to the Safety Assessment
(Toxicity) of Additives by R.D. Combes Ph.D. (Lond.),
M.I.Biol.   294
Appendix II Warning: Dangerous Food Additives —
The Villejuif List   305
Appendix III The Regulation of Food Additives   308
Alphabetical List of Additives and Their E Numbers   317
List of Categories of Food Additives   330
Glossary of Additive Terms   347
References   358
Bibliography   375
Useful Addresses   378
Index   381

Dedication

This new edition is dedicated to:

All those consumers and manufacturers who use the E code wisely to improve the quality of food and of health;

the many scientists, manufacturers and consumers who have provided invaluable technical information;

all those journalists and broadcasters who helped begin a food buying revolution with the first edition;

my patient and dedicated publishers;

my Research Assistant, Jill Marsden, B.Sc., who continues to triumph over the problems of organizing ever increasing quantities of often contradictory scientific information;

the distinguished and still crusading former Minister of Health, David Ennals, for his perceptive and kind foreword;

Leslie Kenton for her foreword to the first edition;

Elizabeth Brown and Angela Beazley for their word-processing skills, often under great pressure;

my family for their support.

Foreword

There has been a revolution in the approach to what we eat. A series of reports have clearly established the link between food intake and health. It has been supported by doctors, pharmacists, dietitians and politicians. In 1985 a decision was made to establish an all-party Parliamentary Food and Health Forum, of which I am Chairman, and this has become one of the most active Parliamentary groups. Across the country there is concern at the fat and sugar content of food and a growing awareness that 30 per cent of adults in Britain are overweight. There is also a growing interest in colourings and artificial flavourings — in fact, in every type of additive. With Britain's appalling record of avoidable diseases, there is now a major campaign linking diet and disease.

This growth in interest has led to a public demand for more information, and since 1962 the EEC has been issuing Directives on additives. Since the beginning of January 1986, most foods have carried a full list of additives, apart from flavourings, described by their E numbers on the package. A great step forward — providing you can fully understand the implication of the E number! For instance, I have aspirin sensitivity, and my wife is asthmatic. So we need to know, for both those conditions tend to bring in their wake sensitivities to certain common food preservatives and colours. The book describes these relationships fully, and in addition makes a convincing case for the full disclosure of ingredients and additives on products where they are not yet required to appear by law, such as in many types of confectionery, alcoholic drinks and medicines.

In 1984, following a great deal of research, Maurice Hanssen's first edition of *E for Additives* was published. It was a tremendous success and was a bestseller for many months, along with Frederick Forsyth and Jeffrey Archer. It is still in great demand. It contains just enough essential information about the contents and effects (including adverse effects) of each product to enable the shopper to know just what they are being asked to buy.

But since 1984, research has provided a mass of additional information about E-numbered additives and about the wider implications of the need for certain additives in foods where many manufacturers are able to produce excellent foods without their use. Key issues such as the nutritional consequences of the over-use of additives are explored for the first time in this new edition of *E for Additives*.

To me, the great merit of Maurice Hanssen's book is that his explanations are clear to all. It is cram full of essential information for the careful shopper. Every essential term, like preservatives, stabilizers, emulsifiers, tenderizers and flavouring, is clearly spelt out.

This book is not just for those who did not buy the first edition. It contains so much that parents need to know. Do additives affect ability, and what about hyperactivity in children? The fact is that more and more is now known about the effects of what we eat — and we *all* need to know.

We *know* that there is a close link between what we eat and our physical — and maybe our mental — health. I doubt whether anyone else in Britain has done more to cut through the commercials and bring out the facts. Maurice Hanssen has been at the forefront of this food and health revolution. For me, it is a real pleasure to commend this new edition. I hope that it, too, will be a bestseller.

THE RT. HON. LORD ENNALS
HOUSE OF LORDS

Foreword to First Edition

This comprehensive book is one which in a sense I wish need never have been written. I would prefer to live in a world where we harvested our foods fresh from the earth, ate them immediately and never had to give a thought to food preservatives, artificial emulsifiers and stabilizers, anti-oxidants and permitted colours. Alas, we do not live in such a world. High technology food production and elaborate chains of food distribution have created a situation in which food additives are necessary. Yet for the protection of oneself and one's family it is also necessary to be well informed about these hundreds of additives in quite specific terms and highly aware of the possible implications of their inclusion in our daily diet.

I therefore welcome Maurice Hanssen's *E for Additives*. Mr Hanssen has produced a simple-to-follow yet remarkably ambitious guide which can help people make informed decisions about the foods on their supermarket shelves even before they buy them. He carefully explains both the pros and cons of food additives, clarifies the meaning of such commonly used but little understood words as 'stabilizers' and 'tenderizers', and offers a quick-to-use guide to each specific additive, its name, where it comes from, the possible adverse effects of using it, and a list of typical products in which it is used. This book is a useful tool for anyone concerned about the health of himself and his family. I for one would not want to be without it.

LESLIE KENTON

Introduction

My first encounter with food additives was in the 1950s when I was concerned with creating new products for people on special diets. It soon became clear to me that many food technologists were using a wide variety of additives simply because they were available, and that they had not really given any thought to the nutritional or health consequences of what they were doing.

I asked the question: 'Why are we using ingredients that I would not need in the kitchen when preparing the same food?' Sometimes there were good technical reasons, but in 90 per cent of the cases there was none. It is because I enjoy cooking at home and because I have a strong background in practical food technology on a factory scale that I began to question whether or not we had true freedom of choice, whether we knew what we were eating and whether many of the additives were necessary at all.

In the 1960s, with the National Association for Health, sponsored by Joyce Butler MP, and with the help of 750,000 well-wishers, we presented a petition to Parliament asking them to 'add all additives'. This was a plea to have a full label declaration of all the ingredients.

For the past 100 or so years there has been an artificial division in our minds between foods and medicines. Since the earliest times man has known that he can live on a wide variety of foods, and that some apparently attractive plants are dangerous whilst some help bring vibrant health and fitness. Even more sophisticated has been the use of very small quantities of otherwise dangerous herbs, such as foxglove or deadly nightshade, which are both still today very important medicines in minute doses.

To stay at the peak of fitness a Roman soldier was only allowed stoneground wholemeal flour. None of the sifted white flour, beloved of the rulers of Rome, found its way into his diet. In the Middle Ages, writers on health said that 'the bread which had all the bran in it was a remedy for constipation caused by eating too much of the fine white bread'! It is obvious that the foods we eat are more important than any additives. But in general terms we have had personal control over our choice of food but little influence on the additives being used.

The 1984 Food Labelling Regulations gave us, for the first time, a good insight into what we were eating and gave me the chance to write *E for Additives*. Even if the book had not sold a single copy I would have needed it for myself and my family. But in the event it was a bestseller which has prompted fundamental changes in the food that we buy. Almost overnight, crisp manufacturers found that they could remove E320 and E321. This may have reduced the shelf-life of the crisps but, with the odd exception of Scotland where apparently food takes a long time to be delivered, the additive-free crisps lasted quite long enough for any shop with a good turnover of stock. This story was repeated, with a wide range of unnecessary and, to some sensitive people, harmful additives, being removed.

A close and careful reading of *The New E for Additives* will show you that there are doubts about only 1 in 5 of the additives commonly used in British food. Some of these have been the most common but, fortunately, public pressure is reducing their usage. Toxicity is dose related and at some level of intake all foods are toxic. We have to keep a balance, but we also have to ensure that we are not being misled with our senses distorted by the use of additives so that high fat and high sugar foods with a very low essential nutrient content give the feeling, appearance, and taste that they are good balanced nutrition. They may be, but an informed look at the label can in most cases give the true picture.

E for Additives provoked a huge correspondence from both consumers and manufacturers, a lot of which was extremely useful in preparing this new edition. It reflects the vast amount of new knowledge that has become available during the intervening three years and its purpose is to increase understanding and to encourage the enjoyment of good, well-prepared foods whether they be in the home, restaurant, health store, or supermarket.

1.
How to Read the Label

Since 1 January 1986 most foods have had to carry a relatively complete list of ingredients. Flavourings do not have to be declared, except by the word 'flavourings', but all the other ingredients, including water, have to be listed in descending order by weight, determined as at the time of their use in the preparation of the food. Water, when there is more than 5 per cent, and other volatile products which are added as ingredients of the food, are listed in order of their weight in the finished product, the weight being calculated in the case of water by deducting from the total weight of the finished product the total weight of the other ingredients used.

If an ingredient used in food is in a concentrated or dried form and becomes reconstituted during the preparation of the food then the weight, in determining the order of the list of ingredients, can be the weight of the ingredient before it has been concentrated or dried. If the food is itself a mixture of concentrated or dried ingredients which have to be reconstituted by adding water, then it is allowable to list the ingredients in descending order of their weight when reconstituted provided that, instead of just saying 'ingredients', the list is preceded by the words 'ingredients of the reconstituted product', or something similar.

If a food consists of, or contains, mixed fruits, nuts, vegetables, spices, or herbs and no particular fruit, nut, vegetable, spice, or herb predominates significantly by weight, the ingredients can be listed in no particular order if the list is headed by a phrase such as 'in variable proportion', and if the variable proportion mix is just a part of the list of ingredients, then the producer can state that that part of the ingredients list is in variable proportion.

Typical Packet Pork Sausages

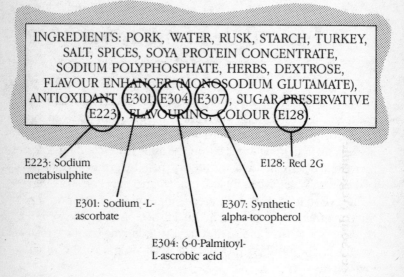

INGREDIENTS: PORK, WATER, RUSK, STARCH, TURKEY, SALT, SPICES, SOYA PROTEIN CONCENTRATE, SODIUM POLYPHOSPHATE, HERBS, DEXTROSE, FLAVOUR ENHANCER (MONOSODIUM GLUTAMATE), ANTIOXIDANT E301, E304, E307, SUGAR PRESERVATIVE E223, FLAVOURING, COLOUR E128.

E223: Sodium metabisulphite

E128: Red 2G

E301: Sodium -L-ascorbate

E307: Synthetic alpha-tocopherol

E304: 6-0-Palmitoyl-L-ascrobic acid

Typical Packet Sliced Meat Loaf (Turkey and Ham)

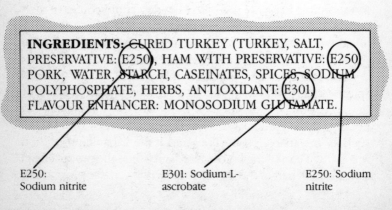

INGREDIENTS: CURED TURKEY (TURKEY, SALT, PRESERVATIVE: E250), HAM WITH PRESERVATIVE: E250 PORK, WATER, STARCH, CASEINATES, SPICES, SODIUM POLYPHOSPHATE, HERBS, ANTIOXIDANT: E301 FLAVOUR ENHANCER: MONOSODIUM GLUTAMATE.

E250: Sodium nitrite

E301: Sodium-L-ascorbate

E250: Sodium nitrite

14

Typical Packet Soup (Vegetable)

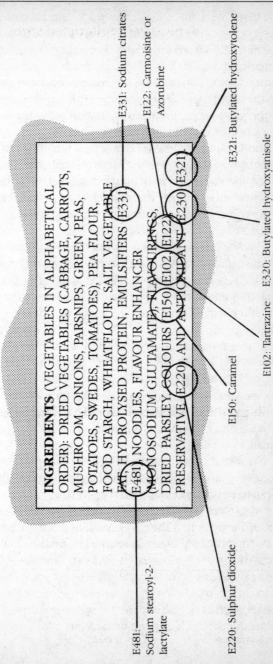

INGREDIENTS (VEGETABLES IN ALPHABETICAL ORDER): DRIED VEGETABLES (CABBAGE, CARROTS, MUSHROOM, ONIONS, PARSNIPS, GREEN PEAS, POTATOES, SWEDES, TOMATOES), PEA FLOUR, FOOD STARCH, WHEATFLOUR, SALT, VEGETABLE FAT, HYDROLYSED PROTEIN, EMULSIFIERS (E481, HYDROLYSED PROTEIN, EMULSIFIERS (E481), NOODLES, FLAVOUR ENHANCER (MONOSODIUM GLUTAMATE), FLAVOURINGS, DRIED PARSLEY, COLOURS (E150, E102, E122), PRESERVATIVE (E220), AND ANTIOXIDANT (E230, E321).

E331: Sodium citrates

E122: Carmoisine or Azorubine

E321: Butylated hydroxytolene

E320: Butylated hydroxyanisole

E102: Tartrazine

E150: Caramel

E481: Sodium stearoyl-2-lactylate

E220: Sulphur dioxide

15

Therefore, with a few exceptions, ingredients are listed in descending order by weight. It is very important to take this into account when reading the label. Many soup or dessert mixes have remarkably similar lists of ingredients in which sugar, starch or flour of some sort, and hydrogenated vegetable fat are high up on the list of ingredients, and sometimes the designated variety of the product such as tomato or strawberry is present in small amounts, or maybe altogether absent.

Food has to be described in a way which is not misleading, using, where there is one, the name prescribed by law, and if there is not, then a customary name, and failing that a precise enough description to inform the purchaser of its true nature and, if needed, a description of its use. A made-up name cannot be used instead of the proper name of the food.

'Flavour' is a word that does not mean quite what it seems to because if a product is, for example, 'strawberry flavour' then it need not contain any strawberry at all. If it is 'strawberry flavoured' then a significant part of its flavour must be from strawberries, and if it is 'strawberry' then it is made with whole strawberries. This is a rule of thumb which is not enshrined in law, and a number of manufacturers and Local Authorities are of the view that both words 'flavour' and 'flavoured' are themselves misleading, and a proper description of the product which does not contain any of the designated substance would be 'artificially flavoured'. Until this is tested in the High Court, or a new regulation is made, the consumer is left with an uncertain and misleading situation.

'No added sugar' is another area of potential misinformation. Because many people are worried that too much sugar will cause them to put on excess weight they look out for products which are sugar-free or contain no added sugar. This description is applied even when the food contains a very large quantity of naturally occurring sugars. An example is jam made without added sugar but with concentrated apple or pear juice containing a naturally high level of sugar. Sugar is being interpreted by certain manufacturers as being just the use of sucrose (table sugar). Other sugars, such as lactose and fructose, are sometimes also included in products which are said to have no added sugar.

Certain diet products are equally misleading; for example, there is a diet bar on sale which has sugar as its second largest ingredient. There is also a tendency for manufacturers to say 'no added colour' or 'no preservatives' or 'no artificial ingredients', all of which may be true but does not alter the fact that the food itself is of low nutritional worth. There is no substitute for reading the ingredient list.

Date Marking

Date marking is now required on most pre-packed foods (with a few exceptions, such as frozen foods, wine and vinegar) unless they have a shelf-life of at least 18 months. Even products with a very long shelf-life may be marked, but this is not mandatory. This is expressed as *either*:

- A best before date (day, month, year) plus storage conditions (if necessary).

Or:

- If the food has a 'life' of between 3 months and 19 months, a best before end date (month, year).
- If the food has a 'life' of between 6 weeks and 3 months, a best before date (day, month) plus storage conditions (if necessary).
- If the food is perishable and is intended for consumption within 6 weeks of being packed, a sell by date (day, month) plus storage conditions and a storage period after purchase.

There is no reason why you should not buy overdue products, especially if they are reduced in price, because the onus is on the shopkeeper to provide goods which live up to the quality of their description, in other words they must not be bad or 'off'. With the longer time datings you are safe in buying goods that are near the end of their expiry date if the shop is clean and well maintained. However if such a product has deteriorated, even if bought at a special price, your legal rights are not affected and you should complain first of all to the shop manager then, if no satisfaction is obtained, to your local Trading Standards Officer, whom you can locate through the Town Hall. It is often preferable, though, to write a nice letter, fully documented, with a sample, to the Managing Director of the company concerned who will often, for the sake of goodwill (and most of the food companies are very jealous of their good reputation), refund your cost and may even give you something extra besides. However, if you are on the make, beware, because most manufacturers keep very accurate records of complainants and get wise to the person who frequently finds a dead mouse in a meat pie.

Foods for special nutritional purposes are subject to the provisions of an EEC Directive which strictly controls all claims and declarations in respect of infant, diabetic, slimming and other foods which purport to be for a group of people with special nutritional needs. There is a problem in that some excellent foods which have a nutritional purpose may not, in the future, be able to declare it without a Medicines Licence! For example, a bran based breakfast cereal may not be able to say that it 'helps constipation', but it can say 'helps to keep you regular' as that is not a medical claim. Too often we are seeing legislation which is designed for consumer protection which effectively shields the consumer from the information needed to make an informed decision. It should surely be sufficient with regard to most claims that labels and advertising are decent, honest and truthful.

Polyunsaturated Fatty Acid Claims
The COMA and NACNE reports on what we should eat for a healthy diet include in their recommendations the view that we should cut down on our total fat intake, have a relatively high proportion of polyunsaturated fatty acids (which are the sort of fats that you have in oils like sunflower, safflower, soya and corn) and consume less animal and dairy fat. This is because such a dietary change is thought to be good for the heart. However, the manufacturer is not allowed by law to tell you that! Before any claims relating to polyunsaturated fatty acids can be made the food has to contain at least 35 per cent of fat by weight. In that fat at least 45 per cent of the fatty acids must be polyunsaturated and not more than 25 per cent saturated.

The claim has to be accompanied by the words 'low in saturates' or 'low in saturated fatty acids' and the food must be marked with a declaration in grammes per 100 grammes or millilitres of the food stating the amount of fat or oil and the amount of polyunsaturated fatty acids (which are cis, cis-methylene interrupted polyunsaturated fatty acids) and also the amount of saturated fatty acids. Each part of the declaration has to be given equal prominence.

If, in addition, the claim is made that it is low in cholesterol, then the food must not contain more than 0.005 per cent of cholesterol and it must be possible to make polyunsaturated fatty acid claims. As in the former case there can be no expressed or implied suggestion that such products are beneficial to health. You have to read the label carefully to see that such a claim is being made if you want to choose truly polyunsaturated margarines such as Flora or, from health stores, the very desirable Vitaquell which contains no animal or dairy ingredients and which has not been hardened by the hydrogenation process.

In the USA sensible and accurate claims for reduced cholesterol foods are allowed as are true statements about the advantages of polyunsaturates. So long as such claims are well controlled they could help many people to change their diet for the better and lessen the risk of heart disease.

Vitamins and Minerals
The Labelling of Food Regulations specify in two schedules the vitamins and minerals for which claims can be made. The word 'claim' has a specific meaning. Vitamins and minerals which are not in the schedule cannot be mentioned at all on a food product except in the nutritional declaration, the name of the product (if it is a food supplement) and the list of ingredients. Anything additional to these three places becomes a claim.

Where it is claimed that the food is a *rich or excellent source* of vitamins or minerals the quantity of food that can reasonably be expected to be consumed in one day must contain at least one half of the recommended daily amount of two or more of the vitamins or minerals in the schedule. Otherwise the claim that the food *contains* the vitamins and minerals can only be made if the quantity of food that can reasonably be expected to be consumed in one day contains at least one sixth of the recommended daily amount of two or more of the vitamins or minerals in the list.

If the claim is confined to named vitamins or minerals then every vitamin or mineral named must be specified in one of the schedules and is then subject to the same requirements as before. The names used in declaring the vitamins must be the names in the first column of the schedules, with or without the words that appear in three cases in brackets.

The names for other vitamins are also specified by law, and are: vitamin B_6, pantothenic acid, biotin, vitamin E and vitamin K. The purpose of this is to prevent people making claims for the existence of vitamins that are not recognized by science, such as vitamin B_{17} and vitamin F.

The following are the two schedules:

Table A

Vitamins in respect of which claims may be made.

Vitamin	To be calculated as	Recommended daily amount
Vitamin A	Micrograms of retinol or micrograms of retinal equivalent on the basis that 6 μg of beta-carotene or 12 μg of other biologically active carotenoids equal 1 μg of retinol equivalent.	750 μg
Thiamin (vitamin B$_1$)	Milligrams of thiamin.	1.2 mg
Riboflavin (vitamin B$_2$)	Milligrams of riboflavin.	1.6 mg
Niacin	Milligrams of nicotinic acid or milligrams of nicotinamide or milligrams of niacin equivalent on the basis that 60 mg of tryptophan equal 1 mg of niacin equivalent.	18 mg
Folic acid	Micrograms of total folic acid.	300 μg
Vitamin B$_{12}$	Micrograms of cobalamines.	2 μg
Vitamin C (ascorbic acid)	Milligrams of ascorbic acid or milligrams of dehydroascorbic acid	30 mg
Vitamin D	Micrograms of ergocalciferol (vitamin D$_2$) or micrograms of cholecalciferol (vitamin D$_3$).	2.5 μg

Table B

Minerals in respect of which claims may be made

Mineral	To be calculated as	Recommended daily amount
Calcium	Milligrams of calcium.	500 mg
Iodine	Micrograms of iodine.	140 µg
Iron	Milligrams of iron.	12 mg

Notes

1. Each vitamin and mineral specified in Tables A and B above includes its biologically active derivative.
2. The quantity of any vitamin or mineral specified in Table A or B above (as extended by note 1 above) shall be calculated in accordance with column 2 of the appropriate Table.

From *Labelling of Food Regulations* No. 1305, 1984.

The idea behind these two schedules was to prevent manufacturers from making claims for vitamins and minerals for which there is no evidence of a shortage. So the schedules represent vitamins and minerals which may be short in the diet and, therefore, all other vitamins and minerals are thought to be present in sufficient quantities in any likely diet. Unfortunately this has led to a very confusing situation, especially with regard to the sale of food supplements such as vitamin, mineral and trace element tablets and capsules which contain either a mixture of scheduled and non-scheduled substances or even exclusively non-scheduled substances. It means that neither in advertising nor on the pack can the manufacturer tell the consumer why the ingredient is there and what it does unless it is on the schedule. A mixture of vitamins A, C and E would therefore have a product description telling you all about vitamins A and C but not saying a single word about vitamin E.

There is much doubt as to whether the list is by any means appropriate to modern day living, and there is increasing evidence that there are substantial groups of people who do not have enough zinc, selenium, magnesium, or vitamins B_6 and E. Groups at risk include children and adolescents on a sugary, fatty diet, and women who take the birth control pill and may need far more B_6 than can be obtained in a likely diet. Unless vegetarians are careful they can be short of zinc, and there is a general shortage of selenium in British soil which used to be supplemented by the use of selenium rich Manitoba wheat for bread making, but now that we make most of our bread from British flour, we could have too little in the diet.

A Committee on the Medical Aspects of Food has been convened under the chairmanship of Dr Roger Whitehead to look at this whole question and suggest a new list of Recommended Daily Amounts, but it is not unreasonable to hope that the position of vitamin and mineral pill manufacturers can be regularized *before* the Committee reports and that regulations can be made so that they are not prevented by law from giving accurate nutritional and biological information about the ingredients to the public — surely an absurd and unnecessary restraint upon our freedom.

What is an Additive?

According to the *Codex Alimentarius*, a food additive is: 'Any substance not normally consumed as a food by itself and not normally used as a typical ingredient of food, whether or not it has nutritive value, the intentional addition of which to food for a technological (including organoleptic) purpose in the manufacture, processing, preparation, treatment, packing, packaging, transport or holding of such food results in, or may be reasonably expected to result (directly or indirectly) in it or its by-products becoming a component of or otherwise affecting the characteristics of such. The term does not include "contaminants" or substances added to food for maintaining or improving nutritional qualities.' ('Organoleptic' means sight, taste, smell and texture as perceived by the senses.)

Because manufacturers can use either the E number or the proper name of the additive as an alternative, they often choose to use the name on the premise that it is less 'frightening' than the E number. On the other hand, some ingredients which have valuable nutritional properties can cause confusion because they have names that look very much like additives, whereas in fact they are not in that class.

A good example is soya protein isolate, which is the valuable protein part of the soya bean in a very pure state and is an extraordinarily good source of very nutritious protein. It can make meat products in particular, such as sausages and pies, as well as a number of other dishes and drinks, more nutritious than they would be without it, and also has useful technical properties in giving the product a better appearance and texture.

Again, if you use an egg yolk because of the emulsifying properties of its natural lecithin then it is declared as the ingredient 'egg-yolk' and not as 'E322', lecithin.

Meat Products

Regulations governing meat products and spreadable fish products were laid before Parliament in October 1984. Like the E-numbering provisions, these came into full operation in July 1986.

Polyphosphates (E450) allow the manufacturer to add water to meat products without it becoming obvious to the consumer.

If the meat is cooked or raw and contains added water, then the producer will have to declare: 'with not more than x per cent added water.' X is the maximum added water content of the food. On the other hand, if the meat is uncooked and cured, such as bacon, of which more than 10 per cent is added water, then the declaration has to say 'with not more than y per cent added water'; but that does *not* mean that this figure represents the amount of added water — y represents a multiple of 5 by which the percentage of water in the product exceeds 10 per cent! Finally, to make matters clear to our (presumably computer owning!) consumer — if it is cooked pure meat then the declaration has to say 'with not more than z per cent added water', z being an indication in multiples of 5 of the percentage of water added.

There is a list of parts of the carcass which may *not* be used in *uncooked* meat products — and may therefore be used in cooked meat products. You will be glad to know what comprehensive use manufacturers of cooked meat products can make of the slaughtered animal; they can use the brains, foot, large intestine, small intestine, lungs, oesophagus, rectum, spinal cord, spleen, stomach, testicles, and udder. There has to be an argument for manufacturers to tell us just what parts of the animal are used and how much, not just to use the blanket description 'offal'.

A meat pie weighing between 100g and 200g must have a meat content of not less than 21 per cent of the total. If the pie weighs less than 100g the meat content can shrink to 19 per cent of the food, otherwise the meat content can soar to the dizzy heights of 25 per cent as a minimum; *but*, of these percentages, the lean meat content need only be half so, at the worst, a quarter of a pound pork pie may contain just over a third of an ounce of lean meat — and it may include unexpected parts of the beast.

The true nature of the contents are then disguised in taste and appearance by the use of flavour enhancers, such as monosodium glutamate (number 621). It can then be coloured, flavoured and, after the addition of the appropriate amount of water, you can have, at the worst, a very fatty pie but one which looks and tastes good. Though of course there are many pie manufacturers who certainly do use the finest ingredients, it would be worth their while making clear claims. The fat content of burgers and sausages is also controlled, in general so that the fat content of the meat part of burgers does not exceed 35 per cent and of sausages, 50 per cent.

Many German meat products are labelled with their fat content. In order to be able to eat sensibly we should demand that such information be available throughout the EEC.

The British government wants to introduce fat content labelling but are being opposed by the EEC. Many responsible food manufacturers are now labelling the fat content voluntarily and this is to be encouraged.

2.
Why Are There Still Secret Ingredients?

The Food Labelling Regulations of 1984 introduced the E-code which made it much easier to identify at least some of the additives in our food. But did they go far enough? There is, in fact, a wide range of foods and other things we swallow where we are not told what the ingredients are.

Alcoholic Drinks

Any drink with an alcoholic strength by volume of more than 1.2 per cent does not have to list the ingredients. This means that if you are, for example, an asthmatic and are particularly sensitive to sulphur dioxide (E220), which is a commonly used preservative in wines, beers and ciders, then you have no way of telling whether it is present or not, let alone whether the content is near the permitted maximum or very low. If you are sensitive then you have to look out for the whole range of sulphites — E220 to 227 — but when the Dutch Consumer Organization tested a selection of wines in 1985, they found that some of them had higher than the permitted limits of sulphur dioxide.

A test published in *Which?* magazine in May 1986 found that a number of the nineteen wines tested were near the maximum and that, if you regularly drank just a quarter litre (2 glasses) of most of the white wines, or one third of a litre (2½ glasses) of some of the reds, you could exceed the Acceptable Daily Intake.

The EEC permits aeration, which is usually done with carbon dioxide (E290), to make cheap sparkling 'bubbly'. To encourage the growth of yeasts during fermentation there is permission for an addition of diammonium phosphate or ammonium sulphate (no E numbers) up to a level of 0.3g/l either separately or combined. You can also feed the yeast by the addition of thiamin hydrochloride (vitamin B_1) up to 0.6mg/l.

The sulphites that may be used include not only sulphur dioxide but also potassium bisulphite and potassium metabisulphite. White wines can be treated during fermentation with charcoal to a maximum of 100g of dry charcoal per hectolitre to remove impurities.

Wine has to be clarified, or cleared, after fermentation. However, some of the ingredients and processing aids that might be used provide significant moral problems for certain sections of the population who surely have the right to know if such items are being included in the process. The full list is:

— edible gelatines (made from bones)
— isinglass (made from the swim-bladders of fish)
— casein and potassium caseinate (milk proteins)
— animal albumin (egg albumin and dried blood powder)
— bentonite (clay) (558)
— silicon dioxide as a gel or colloidal solution (551)
— kaolin (a clay) (559)
— tannin (from wood)
— pectinolytic enzymes.

The use of sorbic acid (E200) or potassium sorbate (E202) is permitted. This stops the growth of yeasts and moulds. The final sorbic acid content of the treated product on its release to the market for human consumption must not exceed 200mg/l.

Tartaric acid (E334) for acidification purposes is permitted, but if there is too much acid, the following may be added under certain conditions:

— neutral potassium tartrate (E336)
— potassium bicarbonate (no E number)
— calcium carbonate (E170) which may contain small quantities of the double calcium salt of L(+)tartaric (E334) and L(−)malic acids (296).

The addition of Aleppo pine resin is permitted, the purpose

being to turn wine into retsina, the typical Greek wine.

L-ascorbic acid (E300) can be added up to 150mg/l and as well as the vitamin C, citric acid can be added for wine stabilization provided that the final content does not exceed 1g/l.

Potassium ferrocyanide (536) can be added to white and rosé wines, as can zinc sulphate heptahydrate (which does not seem to appear on the permitted list) which are used together for 'blue finings'. Red wines can also use calcium phytate (no E number) with up to 100mg/l of metatartaric acid (E353).

Gum acacia (E414) is another permitted additive. DL tartaric acid (E334) precipitates excess calcium, and ion and cation exchange resins can be employed in certain conditions.

Some countries permit the use of discs of pure paraffin impregnated with allyl isothiocyanate (no E number) to create a sterile atmosphere in containers holding more than 20 litres, but there may not be any trace of allyl isothiocyanate in the wine.

Potassium bitartrate (no E number) can be used to assist the precipitation of tartar. The wine can also be treated with up to 20mg/l of copper sulphate (no E number), provided that the copper content in the treated product does not exceed 1mg/l.

So you see that there is more to wine than the simple product of the fermentation of grape juice.

Beer

German beer has traditionally been made from just four ingredients — hops, malt, yeast and water. This was the result of the *Reinheitsgebot*, which was a consumer protection law issued by Duke Wilhelm IV of Bavaria in 1516.

Germany's annual beer consumption is currently 146.5 litres for every man, woman and child. On 12 March 1987 the European Court in Luxembourg overturned the country's decree banning imports of additive-containing beers from other countries. Even Bonn's claim that beer makes up a quarter of the average German man's diet so that the additives could be dangerous to health, did not move the court. It was counter-claimed that when the Germans exported their beer to other countries they were known to put in additives that are not permitted in Germany.

The Germans will go on producing their pure beers for home

consumption and it is quite likely that the many undeclared additives in British beers will effectively deter the German beer drinker from buying them.

In particular, we need to be worried about the substantial additions of caramel (E150), which is the most widely used of all food colours and gives many beers, especially mild, stout, premium bitters, and strong ales, their colour. The 1987 Food Advisory Committee report on colours recommends that there be a maximum content not exceeding 5,000mg/kg, which seems rather high, as the same committee's recommendation for brown bread is a maximum of 2,000mg/kg. Additives in use in beer include agents which keep a good head of froth on the beer and, as in wine, many technical aids, but there is no way of knowing just how 'real' is real ale, let alone the beverages which do not have such honest pretentions. An interesting and effective alternative to caramel is a refined malt. This might be classed as an ingredient rather than an additive.

Other Alcoholic Drinks

Look around any good off-licence and you will see that there must be a very wide variety of colours and additives in use ranging from caramel in whisky to goodness knows what in certain of the more exotic aperitifs and liqueurs. Effectively, there is no regulation whatsoever other than the general provisions of the Food Act.

Unless there is the safeguard of ingredient labelling on alcoholic drinks, disastrous and dangerous episodes such as the Austrian wine scandal — which proved to involve many more countries than just Austria — are certain to happen again. In July 1984 diethylene-glycol was found in Austrian wine in as many as 82 different brands, both in Germany and in Britain. Diethylene-glycol can be used as an anti-freeze, but when added to wine it improves the flavour, so that cheap wines can be sold as superior, more costly products. The expert view is that a consumption of 0.3ml of this contaminant daily is a potential health hazard to the kidneys and that 100ml can be fatal.

A bottle tested in Barnsley was found to contain 1.5ml, and so a heavy drinker could be endangered not only by the alcohol but also by the additive. It is ironic that the only reason the Austrian wine scandal was discovered was that one of the companies using diethylene-glycol in the wine requested a refund of the Value Added Tax. A sharp VAT inspector questioned the large volume of anti-freeze being used in the summer and the scandal was uncovered!

However, the fact is that food inspectors do not generally look very closely at the products which do not have lists of ingredients. Therefore, as things stand, we have very little protection against abuse.

Until public pressure and government action puts this situation to rights there is no reason at all why responsible manufacturers should not voluntarily tell us what is in their drinks. There will be a free, signed copy of this book and a place in history for the first three producers of alcoholic drinks who change their policy by listing all those additives and processing aids in all their products.

Chocolate and Fancy Confectionery

If you pick up a *Mars* bar, you will find that although it lists the percentage of cocoa butter in the chocolate, there is no list of ingredients. This is true of the majority of chocolate confectionery made in the UK, which is, for reasons which are not obvious, excluded from the labelling of ingredient regulations. Perhaps by the time you read this your *Mars* bar will carry a voluntary declaration of ingredients as is the case on some chocolate products.

How can it be that the manufacturers of chocolates with brightly coloured centres that are almost certainly coloured artificially should be allowed to conceal this information? The vast majority of such manufacturers have nothing to hide and everything to gain by telling us all about the good wholesome ingredients that they may be using.

The same lack of information is permitted on fancy confectionery products packed as single items in such forms as a figure, an animal, cigarette, egg, or any other fancy form. Again, some manufacturers tell you what the product is made from. Let us hope the rest follow suit.

Additives in Ingredients and Some Other Exemptions

If an additive has been used in an ingredient which is part of a product containing a number of different ingredients, then the additive does not have to be declared if it serves no significant technological function in the finished product. So, if you buy a breakfast cereal containing apple flakes and the apple flakes look white, this could be because they were carefully processed or it could be because they have an added preservative. There is no way of knowing the difference unless the producer volunteers the information. The same considerations apply to a wide range of foodstuffs.

Bread and Other Fresh Foods

Fresh unwrapped bread carries no list of ingredients simply because there is nowhere to put it. The same applies to cakes and pastries. But when the product is wrapped and sold in an off-the-shelf form, then certain ingredients have to be listed, and you may well find that your wholemeal bread and, even more probably, your brown bread, contains added caramel and numerous other ingredients that are not necessary in the kitchen.

There is no good reason why the foods in the baker's or the butcher's that have been prepared on the premises have no list of ingredients. It would be easy to do and it would help us make an informed choice.

In addition to the unnamed additives on unwrapped bread there are also additives which do not have to be declared even when the product is wrapped. Chief among these must be the flour bleach, benzoyl peroxide (no E number). It is certainly very puzzling that we in Britain need to use a bleach at all when most leading European countries have either banned bleaches or found them completely unnecessary. Another area of contamination is the lingering presence of pesticides and fungicides applied not only to the growing crops but also in the storage silos to prevent insect infestation and fungal growth.

Ham and other meat products on the delicatessen counter have to show the amount of water present (at any rate to some extent, see page 25) but the other additives only need to be identified by their category name, a throw-back to the 1970 regulations. So a ham description may say 'maximum 25 per cent added water, added preservative and colour', unless it is in a packet.

Such loopholes are a negation of all the progress made in other areas of food labelling. The largest part of all food sold in this way is produced by manufacturers who are perfectly able to provide a label for the point of sale giving, in a legible size of lettering, the same information that would be required if the same product were sold in a packet instead of loose, or else it is produced by the shop itself, who must know the recipe.

Even the present very limited regulations are being openly abused in large numbers of shops where no ingredient information at all is supplied about the loose foods on sale. Our Trading Standards Officers, who should be enforcing the rules, have limited resources but are usually most helpful when apparent breaches of the regulations are drawn to their attention. It is a courtesy, however, to first warn the shop management of any likely problem so that they can put things right.

Medicines

A licensed medicine has only to state the details of the active ingredient or ingredients. All the other components of the product are exempt from labelling requirements.

It is not at all uncommon for the good effects of the medicine to be entirely negated by the adverse effects of the other ingredients being used. This is especially true of colours and preservatives. The Ministry of Health, some time ago, distributed a consultative paper to pharmaceutical manufacturers asking them if they would agree to list a limited range of additives which cause side-effects in sensitive people. It is thought that most manufacturers were happy to comply, but no legislation has so far resulted.

In the meantime, the Ministry has said that if you have a problem, all you have to do when buying a medicine is to ask the pharmacist if it has certain ingredients in it. Unfortunately, the pharmacist has no idea because he is not given the information either. He has to go back to the manufacturer who may be unwilling to give him the answer or even to find somebody who has the answer readily available. When the facts emerge they are often disturbing, as in the case of the chewable children's vitamins which contain five different azo-dyes and ground sugar to make them pretty and palatable. There is no reason why pharmaceutical manufacturers should not volunteer to reveal the list of ingredients, and there is no reason why they should be exempted from so doing.

3.
Golden Eggs and Pink-Fleshed Fish

A happy free-range chicken, able to scratch around for its food and choosing many different pigment-containing and mineral-rich items, will usually produce richly golden and strongly shelled eggs. The less fortunate battery hens have to rely upon what is in their feed to give their eggs colour. The most important of these colour-forming substances are, together with other oxygen-containing carotenoids, known by the collective name of xanthophylls (E161).

The xanthophyll content of these fresh feeds is not constant and rapidly degrades during storage periods, so poor colour is a particular problem during the winter months.

Because of the high prices of imported grains compared to those from home, even colour-containing alfafa and maize have been replaced by such cereals as wheat and barley which feed the hens just as well if various fats and soya meals are added, but have no pigments present. A typical laying chicken ration would be as follows:

Wheat	600.00 kg
Extracted soya	155.00
Full-fat soya	50.00
Barley	77.50
Limestone flour	80.00
Fish meal	25.00
Vitamin and trace minerals, calcium and salt	12.50
Total	1000.00 kg

The egg producer studies his market and knows that eggs for table use sell best if the yolks are a nice golden colour, while eggs used for the manufacture of bakery products, pasta and sauces are better yellow.

Egg yolk colours are measured on a scale from pale yellow to deep orange in shades of 1-15. Table eggs are generally at about No. 11 on the scale, although some producers prefer a very deep orange colour for which they demand higher prices. In practice, the feed supplier helps the egg producer choose the desired colour and then adds concentrated red or yellow pigments of synthetic or natural origin to produce the desired effect which is then checked on a regular basis.

It is known that certain free-range egg producers have added naturally occurring pigments to the ration, especially during the cold months, although the legal situation regarding this does not appear to have been established.

Maize-Fed Chickens

In both France and the United States maize-fed or, as the Americans say, corn-fed, chickens with attractive yellow skins are thought to look and taste better than the white birds preferred in Britain, and the colours can be achieved directly from the xanthophylls in the feed. It is possible to cheapen the diet by using a mixture of cereals and supplementing with pigments, or to add pigments to a maize feed to ensure a deep colour.

It is also possible to produce similarly coloured chickens when the feeds are not fresh, and for this purpose lutein (E161b), which can be extracted from marigolds, is added to the feed.

Trout and Salmon

There is a long history of trout farming in Britain, certainly going back to the medieval monasteries where farmed trout brightened the Friday fast. Today the farming of salmon, trout and other fish is big business, but have you ever wondered about the great increase in the availability of delicious pink-fleshed trout and salmon? The pink flesh would, in natural waters, be from fresh foods such as crustaceans, shrimp, prawn, lobster (astaxanthin) and various algae.

It is too expensive to feed the farm fish the crustaceans of their usual environment, so a red pigment, canthaxanthin (E161g), is added to the feed to produce pink flesh. This and certain other pigments, including various forms of carotene and vitamin A, are also sold in tablet form so that we can look as if we have been on a Mediterranean holiday and developed a nice, if often rather yellowish, tan. Be warned though that such coloration gives no protection from sunburn and is there, as in the case of the fish, strictly for appearance's sake.

Other Uses of Pigments

Pigments are commonly found in pet feeds especially for captive birds so that their colourful plumage is maintained. Zoo flamingos are fed with canthaxanthin to ensure the pinkness of their legs, beaks and feathers. Such commonplace pet foods as dog biscuits and meats often appear to contain significant quantities of undeclared colours. It is doubtful whether these are truly appreciated by the animal, but they do attract the owner.

There are widespread abuses of the external colouring of seafood. For example, jumbo prawns and smoked cod's roe are frequently on sale in the fish shop without any ingredient declaration, but they have quite often unquestionably been dipped in a heavy concentration of red dye.

Smoked fish is another loophole. Fish can be called 'smoked' when all that has happened is that they have been dipped in a liquid smoke flavour and then artificially coloured! Indeed, smoked and cured fish which is not packed ready for the consumer, like ham, just has to say 'added permitted colour', but if it is pre-packed the full declaration is required.

Consumer choice means the freedom to make an informed choice, and although we think that the use of these artificial and natural additives in animal feeds presents no toxic hazard to the consumer, we do believe that we have a right, as is the case with eggs in the United States, to know what pigments have been added. In addition, acceptable and legally controlled levels of daily intake should be established and enforced. If the egg regulations are so changed, it would be a good opportunity to label egg boxes with the date the eggs were laid and not the less useful date of packing.

4.
The Colour Problem

Food has been coloured since ancient times. The Romans coloured bread and wine both with 'white earth' and berries. When Britain first imported that rare luxury, sugar, in the twelfth century, the pink- and violet-coloured sugars of Alexandria were, according to John Wallford,[1] great favourites. Tyrian purple (from sea snails), madder (from the roots of a herb) and kermes (from a scale insect) are thought to have provided the varying shades of this part of the spectrum.

The red colour of cochineal (E120), was used at least as early as the tenth century by the Toltecs and then the Aztecs of Central America and, as with Egypt and the Mediterranean countries, where the same dyes were used for cloth and for food, it is most likely that cochineal was a food colour.

Many years ago at social meetings of food chemists and before we were in the least worried about the possibility that sweets could rot the teeth (or to be more precise feed the bacteria that do that dark deed), the manufacturers of *Newberry Fruits*, a range of sweets that were coloured, flavoured and shaped to represent miniature versions of the fruits of which they tasted, gave us a selection of this product in a specially prepared form where all the flavours were jumbled up. Only the most experienced palates could correctly identify a sweet that looked like a strawberry but tasted like a pineapple. So it is clear that colour has a very important role to play in our appreciation and enjoyment of food, affecting not only our eyes but also our taste and even, it is thought, our digestion.

[1] *Historical Development of Food Coloration*, John Wallford. *Developments in Food Colours*, Elsevier 1984.

By the same token, colour can influence us into thinking that inferior food that looks attractive also tastes good and is, no doubt, good for us.

Probably the most widely quoted and, in our view, illogical test of the response of the consumer to colour was undertaken by Dr Nathan Goldenberg of Marks & Spencer following certain complaints that their tinned peas were an artificial shade of green and the strawberry jam was an unnatural red. The colours were removed and the peas became grey/green and the strawberries red/brown. The customers stopped buying and it took a long time with the colours restored to bring back lost sales. The reason why this test was so pointless and inconclusive is that there was no clear explanation to the customers as to why the changes had happened and what they might expect when they took the product home. Today we have a completely different situation where very many manufacturers have taken the green colour out of peas and the red out of strawberry jam and have suffered no loss of sales. This seems to show that, with information and education, we can change our perception as to what looks good and tasty.

Added colour is like a cosmetic. Like all cosmetics colours can improve the appearance, delight the onlooker and deceive the senses. Added colours are not necessary, they are a matter of choice. The author had a letter published in *The Times* on 23 January 1970 which pleaded that, as The World Health Organization had recommended, baby foods should be free from artificial colours, also that we all should be able to tell what is in the food we eat by reading the label. Neither request has yet been granted, but there is hope for babies, for the Food Advisory Committee (FAC) is recommending in its 1987 Report[1] that baby foods should be without artificial colours. We do not know how long it will take to turn this recommendation into law but wish it every success. Only in 1986 did it become necessary to label at least most of the ingredients in the foods that we eat. So the battle to have the freedom to choose what we want to, or do not want to, eat is certainly not quick or easy.

[1] 'Food Advisory Committee Final Report on the Review of the Colouring Matter in Food Regulations 1973', HMSO, 1987.

The Functions of Colours

Colours have well defined food functions:

(a) to reinforce colours introduced into foods by their ingredients but where, without added colouring matter, the colour imparted to the final food by those ingredients would be weaker than the colour the consumer will associate with the food of that type of flavour (e.g. soft drinks, fruit yogurts, pickles and sauces);

(b) to ensure uniformity of colour from batch to batch where ingredients of varying colour intensity have been used (e.g. jams in transparent containers where the customer can compare like with like in the shop);

(c) to restore something of the food's original appearance in those cases where the natural colours have been destroyed by heat processing and subsequent storage (e.g. peas, beans, strawberries and raspberries), or bleached out by the use of preservatives (e.g. fruit preservatives, sulphur dioxide for jam-making out of season), or are not light-stable during prolonged storage (e.g. soft drinks);

(d) to give colour to foods which otherwise would be virtually colourless (e.g. boiled sweets, instant desserts, ice lollies).

'Need' is an essential reason for deciding that a food additive be used. It could be argued that a reasonable response to at least most of the four categories above would be 'needed by whom?'. It is clear that in many cases it is the manufacturer that needs the colour, but as we see the removal of many of the artificial colours from the shelves of our shops it is obvious that more colours are being permitted than are 'needed' by many responsible manufacturers and retailers, and that these are certainly not demanded by us when we have the choice.

Artificial Colours

In the middle of the last century almost anything that gave colour was used to make food products more attractive. Substances containing mercury, lead, cyanide and copper were frequently used. At about the same time in 1856 Sir William Henry Perkin discovered his first 'coal tar dye', which was aniline purple, when he was only nineteen years old. Perkin transformed the cloth industry, whilst at the same time a selection of his colours, which faded less, had a wide range of bright hues and was cheap to use, became available for the food producers.

It did not take long for the regulatory authorities around the world to wonder about some of the colours being used and, depending on where you were, they were either negatively listed, which is to say banned, or positively listed, which means that you could only use those which the government felt were both suitable and harmless according to the scientific standards of the age.

In Britain in 1925 a number of colours which were obviously harmful were banned from use. These included any compounds of antimony, arsenic, cadmium, chromium, copper, lead, mercury and zinc, also one vegetable colour, gamboge (much used by painters), and five of the 'coal tar' colours — picric acid, Victoria yellow, aurine, Manchester yellow and aurantia.

It was not until 1954 that the Food Standards Committee proposed that there should be a list of acceptable colours instead of just a list of those that were not permitted. Accordingly, in both 1957 and 1973 lists of both natural and synthetic colours that were permitted were prepared. So what is the position today? Britain permits more artificial colours than almost any other western country. If Norway can manage without any artificial colours and the United States allows seven, we have to wonder why we permit sixteen.

It must be said that some of them seem to cause very few problems, even in those people who suffer from many allergies and intolerances. The toxicological questions and allergic reactions occur most frequently with E110, sunset yellow, and the yellow colour E102, tartrazine. This could be because they are used quite often. More research is needed, but that which is being undertaken at the moment seems to ignore the well-established fact that many people are allergic or badly affected by both foods and food additives, and that often the combination of the food and the food additive together is worse than either alone.

The 1987 FAC Report has certainly made one major step forward, and that is to give proposed average daily intake upper levels for a number of the colours under review. Very many problems with foods and food additives are related to dose and an effort to reduce the level is welcome. However, the FAC has not looked at the question of need from the consumer's point of view and this could well be an area where the reader will wish to form a personal opinion.

Natural Colours

Professor Frank Curtis, Chairman of the FAC, said in a meeting at the House of Lords in 1987 that he was worried about the increased levels of daily intake of natural colour additives being used, because the tests that had been made on them did not take relatively high levels of consumption into account. This is a fair point. Safety is related to dose. But, having been told that an E-number means that an additive is safe, then it is strange that the natural food colours to do not seem to have been as well tested as we have been led to believe, even though they have received their E-numbers. Nonetheless, so many of them are in common use in a food form that it is difficult to feel really worried about them. For example, if a manufacturer wishes to brighten a strawberry yogurt with beetroot juice instead of E123, amaranth, then the argument goes that the beetroot red colour may also cause problems. On the other hand, beetroot is part of a normal diet whereas amaranth is not.

If we are to be told that colours are necessary for a happy life and a good diet, then certainly a lot more work needs to be done on their safety and necessity, for it is certain that many producers of good food are finding that when they use fine ingredients and first-class methods of conservation the need for colours, artificial or natural, disappears. It is high time we became far less concerned with consistency in the colour of manufactured products, in the way that we do not mind variations of colour in the kitchen. We are already becoming used to a different palette of colours in the foods we eat and this trend will continue as we consume fewer and fewer of those most dispensable of all food additives, the colours.

5.
Flavourings

The Food Act prohibits the addition to food of any harmful substance. Is a flavour harmful or not? — we cannot be sure. The dividing lines between ground almonds, almond essence and synthetic almond flavouring could well illustrate the various stages between being an ingredient and an additive. So it would seem that what we really need to know is precisely what ingredient or additive is being used, so that we have the freedom to decide whether or not to eat it. At the moment there is no statutory declaration of the nature of food flavourings. We also need to have information on the toxicity of these flavours.

The European Community is attempting to produce a framework for controlling flavourings as part of the general harmonization of the Food Law within the community. Because some 4,000 substances are involved this will inevitably take a long time.

Many flavourings are difficult to analyse because they are chemically identical (nature-identical) to the substances which gave the product its character in the first place. This fact could produce bad law because, if you cannot analyse whether the substance is natural or artificial as an additive, then regulations controlling its use have little strength unless we also bring in — and this is envisaged — regular random factory inspections of food manufacturers to check precisely the nature of the ingredients that goes to make up their products. This is in addition to having the contents clearly defined on the label, so that we can make up our minds, too.

The European Community is working towards a positive list, which means giving approval for specified artificial and natural flavours. In spite of obvious difficulties this lack of information remains a substantial gap in our knowledge of what we are eating which should be remedied as soon as possible.

As to safety we have few doubts. Very few problems have been shown to be caused by food flavours and, so far as we can tell, none of these under normal circumstances. This is because the effectiveness of a food flavour depends on it being chemically similar to that found in nature and, if you happen to be allergic to strawberries, you would be unlikely to eat strawberry-flavoured products which could produce the same problems.

Watch out for 'smoked' fish. It is legally permissible to dip fish into 'liquid smoke', which is in truth a flavour, and then add colour as a replacement for the hues of the normal smoking process. Such fish can be described as 'smoked'. Also, both smoked and cured fish, as with ham, when sold not ready-packed only have to carry the words 'added permitted colour', and so avoid the obligation to give a true list of ingredients.

6.
P for Pesticides

A report from the American National Academy of Sciences was stated, according to an article in *The Independent* of 28 May 1987, to have studied 28 of the 53 pesticides which the Environmental Protection Agency deemed to be carcinogenic.

There was a lack of data on a number of the other pesticides used, but it was found that a small number of the widely used pesticides posed the greatest hazard to health, and it was suggested that three petrochemical compounds — the herbicide linuron and the insecticides chlorodineform and permethrin — be banned.

Permethrin is sprayed on almost every fruit, nut and vegetable purchased in America, says the article, and linuron is extensively used on soya beans and potatoes.

The difficulty for the EPA, which is a government agency, is that if it bans a chemical as being harmful to the consumer then it has to pay the manufacturer the cost of all the unused chemical plus the anticipated margin of profit.

It has frequently been suggested that we write a book as informative about pesticides as we hope this is about additives. The difficulty is clear. You cannot tell if a product contains an excessive quantity of pesticides without a clear labelling obligation. Until this comes about all that can be done is to give general guidance.

The Americans came to the conclusion that, if the fruits and vegetables are sprayed with the worst possible selection of permitted pesticides, the rating list of danger from contracting cancer was:

Tomatoes, beef, potatoes, oranges, lettuce, apples, peaches, pork, soya beans, wheat, beans, carrots, chicken, grapes and corn.

As to risk, the committee thought that 5.8 cases of cancer per thousand people consuming this list of foods when treated with the pesticides specified was a realistic forecast. There can be no better argument for selecting organically grown fruit and vegetables with some seal of approval — the most reliable being that of the Soil Association — and also dairy products and meat with similar quality controls. Fortunately, this branch of farming which was pioneered by the health food suppliers has now spread into a wider market and you should look out for 'organic' signs on foods which will not only have very low levels of pesticides but also very superior flavour.

Foods, herbs and spices, imported from overseas are rarely checked for pesticide residues. Those tests that have been undertaken show very grave cause for concern.

For example, lettuces from certain Mediterranean growers are produced in polythene tunnels under a continual mist of insecticides, fungicides and water until the moment of picking. The laboratory equipment at our ports is so out-dated that 10-14 days are required for analyses by which time the food would be bad. Finland has achieved the highest standards for import quality control, possibly the best in the world, with the result that growers produce special low pesticide residue produce for that country. We must demand equal standards throughout the EEC.

7.

Is It Kosher?

Certain religious disciplines, such as those of the Jews, the Muslims and the Sikhs, as well as those who have an ethical objection to certain foods or additives, have written us many letters asking distinctions to be made between additives that are animal, dairy, vegetable and synthetic. In addition, synthetic additives can be made from natural materials. Wherever possible this information is included in this edition, but there are a number of cases where the additive can be derived in different ways, some of which would be acceptable to particular groups and some of which would not.

This gives rise to the apparent paradox that some foods are approved by the Rabbinical authorities but contain additives which are on the banned list. In all cases this means that the food has been checked back to source, additives and all, and it has been prepared in accordance with Jewish principles.

List of non-kosher food additives:

E120	E422	430	431
432	433	434	435
436	E470	E471	E472(a)
E472(b)	E472(c)	E472(e)	E473
E474	E475	476	E477
478	E481	E482	E483
491	492	493	494
495	542	570	572
904			

Additives, or ingredients, which have not been allocated EEC numbers, and may also be derived from non-kosher sources, are:

Edible fat or oil; gelatin; enzymes of catalase, lipase, pepsin, trypsin and rennin (or rennet); modified starch with glycerol; glyceryl tribenzoate, glyceryl tributyrate and glyceryl tripropionate; glycine; oxystearin; stearic acid and stearates; monoacetin, diacetin and triacetin; spermacetti; sperm oil; casein and caseinates; wine vinegar; wine or brandy as flavouring agents; proteins.

Note that whey and lactose are milk derivatives. Please note also that the additives and processing aids used in wine making, and therefore also in the preparation of fortified wines such as sherry and in brandies, are frequently of animal or dairy origin. These would normally be removed before the wines are bottled. In both this case and for the additives listed above, where there is any doubt it would be a simple matter for the regulations to be changed so that, for example, an (A) was used as a suffix for additives which were derived from animal material and the suffix (D) for those from dairy material.

It would unquestionably be fruitful for there to be a coming together of the leaders of the many groups involved, including vegetarians, vegans, Jews, Muslims, Sikhs, Hindus, Buddhists and Seventh Day Adventists, who would certainly together form a sufficiently persuasive and numerically strong grouping to convince both the British Ministry of Agriculture, Fisheries and Food and also the EEC Commission in Brussels that such additive identification is both necessary and possible. As things stand, the problem is hardly recognized as existing.

8.
Do Additives Affect Ability?

New York City State schools have some of the highest paid and best qualified teachers in the USA yet in the late 1970s they had some of the worst records of academic success and criticism of both pupils and teachers was reaching a desperately high level. What could be done?

Dr Elizabeth Cagan, a distinguished and charismatic educationalist, was routed out from her academic environment and given the challenge of reforming the school catering service, because it was felt instinctively that this could be part of the problem.

Liz Cagan looked at the food served to the children and said to herself that this was far removed from the plain, sensible, nourishing food which she had served to her own family. Aircraft-type meals were warmed up and most of them finished up in the rubbish bin. She called the cooks together and told them that, if they were to stay in work, they had to become real cooks and not just re-heaters.

Not long after, through one of her assistants, she heard of the pioneering experiments of Alexander G. Schauss, a brilliant penologist, who had turned to biosocial research and nutrition. He had experimented with prison populations by giving them food low in additives and sugar. There had been substantial improvements in work records and less aggression. In Alabama, for example, after a control period of 18 months without diet modifications, a revised diet was introduced. Within 4½ months of changing the diet policy behaviour problems fell and then levelled off for the next 14 months of the trial at a figure 61 per cent lower than before.

These results were validated by a number of other controlled trials where the data confirmed that diet and behavioural problems have many cause-and-effect links, and these included problems with sugar, food colours and, indeed, flavours.

The Feingold Diet, which was on the same basic lines with also the removal of the antioxidants BHA and BHT (E320 and E321), had produced successful results with both hyperactivity and juvenile delinquency.

So, Dr Cagan's colleague went to see Alexander Schauss and between them they decided to set up a food system for the New York City schools which, incidentally, have the second biggest buying power for food products after the US Army, in a first-phase Feingold Diet. This involved a gradual elimination of artificial colours, artificial flavours and the preservatives BHA and BHT while, simultaneously, foods high in sugar were either eliminated or the sugar reduced to a maximum figure of around 11 per cent.

It was ensured that, when each revision was implemented, changes took place simultaneously in all the schools, but the revisions were carried out over three academic years: 1979–80, 1980–81 and 1982–83, with no changes being made in the 1981–82 academic year so that there was a basis for evaluating the effects of change.

All the selected schools gave their children the California Achievement Test (CAT), which is given to many schools across the United States and from which the percentage ranking of the school was calculated.

They had already checked back for the four years preceding the changes so that they knew the average figures involved: these did not fluctuate by more than a mere percentage point. The mean academic CAT score for each school was calculated and then it was converted to a national ranking by comparing this mean with that of the other schools who used the same test in the same year. Then the previous year's ranking was subtracted from the current year's to show the gain or loss in national terms. The figures for all 803 schools averaged together show a mean gain or decline in the years between 1977 and 1983.

This exceptionally complex trial on almost a million children who ate both breakfast and lunch at school was undertaken by three doctors, Stephen J. Schoenthaler, Walter E. Doraz and James A. Wakefield Jr. It was published in the *International Journal of Biosocial Research*, Volume 8, Number 2, 1986, pp.138-148.

The results were astounding. There was a 15.7 per cent increase in mean academic ranking over and above the rest of the nation's schools who used the same standardized tests. (Before the changes the variations had been less than 1 per cent.) Prior to dietary changes, the school children who ate the most school meals had the worst results. After the changes, the children who ate the most school meals had the best results. Never before had there been a trial of such a size and with such scientific support on so many children to determine the effect of diet upon ability.

The schools formed committees including pupils to set up their own menus, along Dr Cagan's guidelines, with their cooks and dieticians. There were supportive posters everywhere such as 'Have you hugged your dietician today?' (which in some areas was altered by changing the h to m!). When Dr Cagan went to a school in the roughest part of New York City and was introduced at meal time by the head teacher as being the lady who had changed the food, she received a standing ovation from the pupils. Only a few years before, visitors would have required a police escort.

So, do certain additives damage the brain? We do not know. What does look certain from this gigantic and extraordinary trial is that there has to be a reconsideration of those additives which deny children the nutrients normally present in real food.

What is the purpose of excessive quantities of sugar, colours, flavours and preservatives? They are there to disguise nutritionally unimportant food substances, including highly calorific fats, as real, wholesome, satisfying food. Just go round your supermarket and look at the foods still being sold that appeal to the senses of the young. Without checking the labels carefully you can easily buy non-nutritive rubbish. But it tastes and looks just like real food. So additives can dilute nutrition. The test of 'need' is applied without a true understanding of the consequences to our children, upon whom all our future hopes must be founded.

Remember, many additives help to provide us with good and safe food, but beware — additives that in themselves might be harmless deceive us and, worse still, our children, into consuming empty calories.

* * * * *

A centre for severely disturbed children — the state-run Aycliffe School in Co. Durham — is undertaking a trial to find whether the Schauss/Schoenthaler Diet, which they will be adapting, can help these children.

The diet being used observes the following guidelines:

(a) sweetened breakfast cereals to be replaced with non-sweetened varieties;

(b) canned fruits, if packed in syrup, to be rinsed with cold water before serving;

(c) soft drinks to be replaced with a wide selection of fruit and vegetable juices;

(d) table sugar to be replaced with honey;

(e) wholemeal bread to be substituted for white bread;

(f) brown rice to replace white rice;

(g) processed foods to be replaced with fresh, when available at similar prices;

(h) snack foods high in sugar, fat or refined carbohydrates to be replaced by fresh fruit and vegetables, plus a variety of nuts, cheeses and wholegrain biscuits;

(i) preservatives, especially BHA (E320) and BHT (E321), and artificially coloured or flavoured foods to be avoided where possible.

In this special group of children the results may not necessarily be generally applicable, but they will be of great importance. Further studies need to be done.

9.
Hyperactivity in Children

A lot of cynicism has been generated about the whole idea of hyperactivity in children. 'There are no hyperactive children, only hyperactive parents' is a frequent retort. The evidence is mounting, although with some reservations, that a good deal of so called hyperactivity is, in fact, due to an unstable environment, but that a good deal is due to food. Dr Egger at Great Ormond Street Hospital showed in his series of cases that there were no children who had an adverse effect from additives only. They were always affected by a food as well.

Dr Ben Feingold MD began his work and observations in 1965 on the link between certain foods and additives and the effect on some individuals' behaviour and their ability to learn. He proposed a diet which cut down on certain additives and eliminated certain foods. Scientific workers are still uncertain as to the validity of the whole of Dr Feingold's ideas, but there is no doubt that a vast number of hyperactive children, and also asthmatics and those suffering from eczema, have benefitted immeasurably from a sensible and careful adaptation of this diet.

Hyperactive children bring much strain and exhaustion to parents who have to manage offspring who only sleep a few hours; are excitable and impulsive; are very fidgety; have a short attention span; are compulsively aggressive; can hurt themselves and are sometimes very anti-social. All these traits are beyond the control of the children, who may well also suffer from a lack of co-ordination of the muscles. They collide with objects when trying such simple sports as cycling and swimming. Their finer senses, such as their eyes and hands, do not seem to operate together. They have difficulty with buttoning and tieing, writing, drawing and speaking — sometimes they are dyslexic.

As they grow older they become even more active and can easily hurt. Difficulties are experienced with speech, balance and learning, even if the IQ is high. They suffer from excessive thirst and are often prone to respiratory difficulties.

It was to help such parents and children that the Hyperactive Children's Support Group was formed in 1977. It is now a registered charity. The Secretary is Mrs Sally Bunday, 71 Whyke Lane, Chichester, West Sussex PO19 2LD (please enclose an SAE if you would like details of membership). The Group recommends that parents try a diet based on the work of Ben Feingold. First, this means cutting out all food and drink containing synthetic colours or flavours, avoiding glutamates, nitrites, nitrates, BHA, BHT and benzoic acid. Second, for the first four to six weeks, foods containing natural salicylates (like aspirin chemically) should be avoided and then re-introduced one at a time to see if they cause problems. Such foods include almonds, apples, apricots, peaches, plums, prunes, oranges, tomatoes, tangerines, cucumbers, most soft fruits, cherries, grapes and raisins.

The additives that the HACSG recommends should be avoided are:

E102	Tartrazine
E104	Quinoline Yellow
107	Yellow 2G
E110	Sunset Yellow FCF
E120	Cochineal
E122	Carmoisine
E123	Amaranth
E124	Ponceau 4R
E127	Erythrosine
128	Red 2G
E132	Indigo Carmine
133	Brilliant blue FCF
E150	Caramel
E151	Black PN
154	Brown FK
155	Brown HT

E160(b)	Annatto
E210	Benzoic acid
E211	Sodium benzoate
E220	Sulphur dioxide
E250	Sodium nitrite
E251	Sodium nitrate
E320	Butylated hydroxyanisole
E321	Butylated hydroxytoluene

Plus another antioxidant preservative not used in the UK

TBHQ	(Monotertiary butylhydroxylquinone)

Additives which are either dangerous to asthmatics or aspirin-sensitive people, and could reasonably be added to the HACSG listing, or should not be used in food intended for babies or young children are:

E212	Potassium benzoate
E213	Calcium benzoate
E214	Ethyl 4-hydroxybenzoate
E215	Ethyl 4-hydroxybenzoate, sodium salt
E216	Propyl 4-hydroxybenzoate
E217	Propyl 4-hydroxybenzoate, sodium salt
E218	Methyl 4-hydroxybenzoate
E219	Methyl 4-hydroxybenzoate, sodium salt
E310	Propyl gallate
E311	Octyl gallate
E312	Dodecyl gallate
621	Sodium hydrogen L-glutamate (*mono*Sodium glutamate)
622	Potassium hydrogen L-glutamate (*mono*Potassium glutamate)
623	Calcium dihydrogen di-L-glutamate (calcium glutamate)
627	Guanosine 5'-(*di*Sodium phosphate)
631	Inosine 5'-(*di*Sodium phosphate)
635	Sodium 5'-ribonucleotide

The medical profession still believes that more work is needed with larger trials, but in the meantime such diets are very valuable if you, having adopted them, then reduce the number of forbidden substances and foods so that the child concerned is left with as large a variety as possible, is not kept out of the main stream of childhood fun, and does not suffer from unnecessarily restrictive rules.

10.
The Avoidable 57 Additives

Additives can hide the true nature of food. You can use polyphosphates (E450) to emulsify fat and to incorporate water, some 128 (Red 2G) to colour the fat so that it looks like meat, enhance the flavour with 621 (monosodium glutamate), so that the food has an addictive and chicken-like flavour. Add some BHA and BHT, E320 and E321, to make sure that the excessive quantities of fat do not go rancid, mix in some lean meat and salt, and surround the mixture with a pastry of white flour and lard, then you have a meat pie which contains very little lean fleshed meat and lots of the sort of saturated fat that our government advises us to eat only in moderation. The additives make sure that our senses do not detect the fat.

What are the most unnecessary or potentially worrying additives? That list only contains some 1 in 5 of those with numbers. These 57 different substances, with rather more chemical names, are:

E102	Tartrazine
E104	Quinoline yellow
107	Yellow 2G
E110	Sunset yellow FCF
E120	{ Carmine of Cochineal Carminic acid Cochineal
E122	{ Azorubine Carmoisine
E123	Amaranth
E124	Ponceau 4R

E127	Erythrosine
128	Red 2G
E131	Patent blue V
E132	Indigo carmine
133	Brilliant blue FCF
E142	Acid Brilliant Green Green S Lissamine Green
E150	Caramel
E151	Black PN
E153	Carbon black Vegetable carbon
154	Brown FK Food Brown Kipper brown
155	Brown HT Chocolate brown HT
E173	Aluminium
E180	Lithol Rubine BK
E210	Benzoic acid
E211	Sodium benzoate
E212	Potassium benzoate
E213	Calcium benzoate
E214	Ethyl-4-hydroxybenzoate Ethyl para-hydroxybenzoate
E215	Ethyl-4-hydroxy-benzoate, sodium salt
E216	Propyl 4-hydroxybenzoate
E217	Propyl 4-hydroxybenzoate, sodium salt
E218	Methyl 4-hydroxybenzoate, sodium salt Methyl para-hydroxybenzoate
E219	Methyl 4-hydroxybenzoate, sodium salt
E220	Sulphur dioxide
E221	Sodium sulphite
E222	Sodium bisulphite Sodium hydrogen sulphite
E223	Sodium metabisulphite
E224	Potassium metabisulphite
E226	Calcium sulphite

E227	Calcium bisulphite
E250	Sodium nitrite
E251	Sodium nitrate
E310	Propyl gallate
E311	Octyl gallate
E312	Dodecyl gallate
E320	{ BHA Butylated hydroxyanisole
E321	{ BHT Butylated hydroxytoluene
385	{ Calcium *di*Sodium EDTA Calcium *di*Sodium ethylenediamine-NNN'N' tetra-acetate
E407	Carrageenan
E450	Polyphosphates
621	{ *mono*Sodium glutamate MSG Sodium hydrogen L-glutamate
622	{ *mono*Potassium glutamate Potassium hydrogen L-glutamate
623	{ Calcium *di*hydrogen di-L-glutamate Calcium glutamate
627	{ Guanosine 5' (disodium phosphate) Sodium guanylate
631	{ Inosine 5' (disodium phosphate) Sodium 5' inosinate
635	Sodium 5'-ribonucleotide
924	Potassium bromate
925	Chlorine
926	Chlorine dioxide

Sodium nitrate and sodium nitrite, E250 and E251, are in this list because there is evidence that links them with producing carcinogenic nitrosamines. But the use of nitrates and nitrites in the preservation of cured meats is long established and prevents, among other things, the growth of the lethal botulinum.

The potassium salts of nitrates and nitrites, E249 and E252, are not included in the list, although they are also problematical, as it is recognized that chemical means to preserve meat are, at this time, necessary. They have the advantage of not adding to the amount of sodium in the diet.

What is included in any list of avoidable additives is a personal decision and the wise approach is to make your own list.

11.
The Natural Opportunity for Profit

The food revolution following the publication of *E for Additives* produced two conflicting results. The first was a whole lot of foods that were nutritionally better as well as being free from unnecessary and possibly harmful additives. The second was the use of such statements as 'free from artificial colours' and others, including the frequent use of the word 'natural' to give the impression that the food was just as if it had been taken from an old world farm and prepared specially for you with the care and consideration of a good home cook. These foods are taking a step along the right road but you have to be very discriminating indeed.

If a product says 'no artificial colourings', then that is all very well but what are the other ingredients? The overall concept of a healthy and balanced diet is far more important than any concern you may have for the odd E-additive unless you have a special sensitivity. It is the food we eat that makes us fit and healthy and the trick is to avoid being misled by advertising and pack presentation which makes you think that the absence of certain ingredients means that by default other good nutritional substances must be there. They may, but there again they may not.

The E-code has given us the freedom to make informed decisions about some of the foods we eat, but those decisions should not just be based on the additives but upon the whole nutritional concept of the food. On the other hand, food is also fun, and if you like to enjoy a few potato crisps, that is just fine. It is truly an advantage that you can now obtain them without BHA and BHT (E320 and E321), with natural flavours, and cooked in vegetable oil.

The food industry has to make a profit in order to survive and to have the money available to develop new and interesting foods. It is our job to make sure that the promises on the packet are supported by the composition of the product; for by selecting for our personal use those products which are truly honest and nutritionally sensible and, not to be forgotten, taste good, we shall be supporting those manufacturers, and there are many of them, who truly understand the difference between nutritional hype and nutritional help.

12.
The E Number Categories

E100   **Curcumin (C.I. 75300)**

Source   Extract of dried rhizome of *Curcuma longa*
                  (turmeric), a member of the ginger family, grown
                  in India, West Pakistan, China and Malaya. The
                  lateral rhizomes contain the most colouring
                  materials, known as curcuminoids. Curcumin, the
                  pure colouring principle of the spice turmeric,
                  is obtained by solvent extraction of turmeric using
                  methanol, hexane and acetone.

Function   Water soluble orange-yellow colour. Used in
                  many new products as a replacement for artificial
                  colours.

Effects   There were no adverse effects seen in rats and
                  mice fed 0.1 per cent curcumin over 90 days, but
                  the thyroid weight of pigs increased when fed
                  60-1550mg/kg body weight curcumin for over
                  100 days, and the thyroid cells multiplied
                  abnormally. Long-term studies in rats are in
                  progress to try to help understand these results.

A.D.I.   0–0.1mg/kg body weight (temporary to 1987).

Typical Products	Edible fats and oils to restore colour lost in processing
	Savoury rice
	Flour confectionery
	Curry powders
	Margarine
	Processed cheese
	Butter
	Ice cream
	Fish cakes and fish fingers
	Chicken pies

E101   Riboflavin (Lactoflavin; Vitamin B$_2$)

Source

Occurs naturally in liver, kidneys, green vegetables, malted barley, eggs and milk, and a small amount is synthesized by bacteria in the large intestine. Manufactured from yeast or other fermenting organisms, such as *Ashbya gossypii* or *Eremothecium ashbyii*, or more often by synthesis starting with O-xylene, D-ribose or alloxan.

Function

Yellow or orange-yellow colour; vitamin B$_2$. Has poor solubility, so is difficult to incorporate into many liquid foods, and is also sensitive to light.

Effects

Little riboflavin is stored in the body; excess of requirements is excreted in the urine. No toxicological problems even with intakes far exceeding the nutritionally required levels. There is a suggestion that riboflavin in the diet may prevent the reduction of azo dyes (see glossary) by intestinal bacteria.

A.D.I.

0–0.5mg/kg body weight. The levels in foods intended for babies and young children are limited to the amounts used as a vitamin supplement.

Typical Products	Sauces
	Processed cheese
	Pickled cucumbers
	Vitamin enrichment
	Milk products, condensed or dried
	Foods described on the label directly or by implication as being specially prepared for babies or young children limited to amounts permitted in vitamin supplements as a medicine.

101(a)   Riboflavin-5'-phosphate (Riboflavin-5'-[Sodium phosphate])

Source   Prepared by chemical action on riboflavin (E101). Riboflavin-5'-phosphate consists mainly of the monosodium salt of the 5'-monophosphate ester of riboflavin dihydrate.

Function   Yellow or orange-yellow colour; vitamin B_2 — a more soluble form of riboflavin, but also more expensive.

Effects   The phosphate is rapidly hydrolysed after ingestion to yield riboflavin. Riboflavin and riboflavin-5'-phosphate are in metabolic equilibrium after absorption. There are no toxicological problems with riboflavin even when taken in amounts far exceeding the nutritionally required levels or any likely food use.

A.D.I.   0–0.5mg/kg body weight (temporary).

Typical Products   The levels in foods intended for babies and young children are limited to the amounts used as a vitamin supplement.
Various sugar products

Jams
Milk products, condensed or dried
Under consideration by the EEC for an 'E' prefix.

E102   **Tartrazine (C.I. 19140: FD and C Yellow 5)**

Source   Synthetic, an azo dye (see glossary).

Function   Yellow colour.

Effects   Tartrazine appears to be the most reactive of all the azo dyes. In a double-blind crossover placebo-controlled trial with 76 selected overactive children, tartrazine and benzoic acid (E210) provoked a response in 79 per cent of those tested but no child reacted to either substance individually.

In a study of 88 children with severe frequent migraine headaches tartrazine caused symptoms in 12 of them.

Tartrazine provokes a response in some adult asthmatics, particularly those sensitive to aspirin, although aspirin-intolerant people are not necessarily intolerant to tartrazine. It also makes the condition worse in between 10 and 40 per cent of patients with chronic urticaria (nettle rash), and possibly intensifies the reactions of a higher proportion still of aspirin-sensitive individuals. However, the 1987 Food Advisory Committee's report on the Colouring Matter in Food Regulations states that placebo-controlled provocation studies are shedding doubt on the aspirin/tartrazine association and the matter is as yet unresolved. The Hyperactive Children's Support Group recommends that this colour, among others, be eliminated from the diets of the children it represents.

Other adverse reactions in susceptible people include itching, rhinitis (runny nose), blurred vision, and purple patches on the skin, and it has been suggested that tartrazine in fruit flavour cordials may be responsible for wakefulness in small children at night.

There appears to be no clear scientific explanation of how tartrazine causes a response in sensitive individuals. Some reactions, because they happen quickly on low doses, suggest an allergy. Tartrazine has been shown to raise the plasma histamine levels of normal healthy adults when large doses of more than 50mg are given. Skin tests with tartrazine, however, often fail to produce a reaction, so it may mean that a breakdown product of tartrazine is responsible.

An accurate assessment of tartrazine sensitivity in the general population can be only a guess. One source (BIBRA) supposes that 0.06–0.24 per cent of the population as a whole might be sensitive to tartrazine. This would represent between 34,000 and 134,000 people in the UK. Survey work undertaken on behalf of the Ministry of Agriculture, Fisheries and Food suggests that intolerance to *all* food additives is something approaching 0.4 per cent (or 222,000) of the population.

A.D.I.	0–7.5mg/kg body weight.

Typical Products	Fruit squash and cordial Coloured fizzy drinks Instant puddings Packet convenience foods Cake mixes

Custard powder
Soups (packets and tins)
Bottled sauces
Pickles
Salad cream and salad dressings
Ice cream and lollies
Sweets
Chewing gum
Marzipan
Jam
Marmalade
Jelly
Smoked cod and haddock
Mustard
Yogurt
Shells of medicinal capsules
Glycerin, lemon and honey products

A very commonly used colour. Its use is prohibited in Norway and Austria.

E104   **Quinoline Yellow (C.I. 47005)**

Source   Synthetic 'coal tar' dye (see glossary), the disodium salt of disulphonic acid. There are two quinoline yellows, the so-called 'earlier' and 'later' quinoline yellows; the latter is about 30 per cent methylated, the former is non-methylated.

Function   Dull yellow to greenish-yellow colour.

Effects   Short-term studies of quinoline yellow in dogs and rats showed that the dye was poorly absorbed from the food canal. There were no dose-related effects following a three generation study in the rat and a long-term/carcinogenicity study in the mouse was satisfactory. On this basis the Food Advisory Committee recommended that the use of quinoline yellow in food was acceptable. It is one of the colours which the Hyperactive Children's Support Group recommends should be eliminated from the diet of the children it represents.

A.D.I.   0–0.5mg/kg body weight.

Typical   Scotch eggs
Products   Smoked haddock
                 Ices and ice mixes
                 Its use is prohibited in Norway, the United States,
                    Australia and Japan.

---

107   **Yellow 2G (Food Yellow 5)**

Source   Synthetic 'coal tar' dye, and azo dye (see glossary).

Function   Food colour.

Effects   Yellow 2G belongs to a group of chemical dyes known as azo dyes. People who suffer from asthma and those sensitive to aspirin may also show an allergic reaction to this colour. It is one of the food colours which the Hyperactive Children's Support Group recommends should be eliminated from the diet of the children it represents.

A.D.I.   No A.D.I.

Typical   The EEC is proposing the total banning of Yellow
Products   2G. Once this proposal is accepted the
                 marketing of foods containing it will be
                 prohibited 18 months following notification.

The Food Advisory Committee have recommended that Yellow 2G should be withdrawn from use in Britain.

Within the EEC the UK is the only country to retain its use. It is banned in Norway, Sweden, Austria, Switzerland, Japan and the United States.

E110 Sunset Yellow FCF (C.I. 15985; FD and C Yellow 6)

Source Synthetic 'coal tar' dye, and azo dye (see glossary).

Function Yellow colour, especially useful for fermented foods which must be heat-treated.

Effects An azo dye to which some people have an allergic reaction. Hypersensitivity may occur especially in people showing aspirin sensitivity, producing urticaria (nettle rash), angioedema (swelling on the skin), gastric upset and vomiting. It is one of the food colours which the Hyperactive Children's Support Group recommends should be eliminated from the diet of the children it represents.

The dye is minimally absorbed in rats, mice, guinea pigs, rabbits and man, and is able to cross the placenta.

In 1984 animal studies in the United States showed this dye to be weakly carcinogenic. These results are not, however, consistent with other work with rats and mice.

In view of all the results, the Food Advisory Committee did not consider the findings in the recent experiments attributable to Sunset Yellow FCF and are happy with its continued use as a food colour.

A.D.I.   0–2.5mg/kg body weight.

Further studies by the Joint FAO/WHO Expert Committee on Food Additives reduced the recommended acceptable daily intake level by 50 per cent in 1982.

Typical Products

Hot chocolate mix
Packet soup
Sweets
Packet trifle mix
Yogurts
Yogurt whip
Packet sorbet mix
Orange jelly biscuits
Packet breadcrumbs
Packet cheese sauce mix
Orange squash
Marzipan
Swiss roll
Apricot jam
Citrus marmalade
Lemon curd
Tinned shrimps and prawns
Tinned apple sauce
Pickled cucumbers
Ices and ice mixes

Its use is prohibited in Norway and Finland.

E120   Cochineal (Carmine of cochineal; Carminic acid; C.I. 75470; Natural Red 4)

Source   Cochineal is the natural red colour which accumulates in the bodies of pregnant scale insects (*Dactilopius coccus* (Dactilopiidae)). The insects breed and feed on particular cacti (species of Nopalea) and both are indigenous to Central America. Commercial supplies are obtained from

Peru, the Canaries, Algiers and Honduras. The extract contains about 10 per cent of carminic acid. Carmine is produced from cochineal, as is aluminium lake. Both cochineal products contain aluminium complexes of carminic acid.

Function Expensive but effective red colouring for liquids and (ammonium carmine) solids, indicators and diagnostic agents. The water-soluble form is used exclusively for colouring alcoholic drinks; the insoluble form (calcium carmine) has wider colouring applications.

Effects This is one of the food colours which the Hyperactive Children's Support Group recommends should be excluded from the diet of children it represents. A long-term carcinogenicity study on the liquid form of cochineal in rats showed no carcinogenic or other adverse effects.

A.D.I. 0–2.5mg/kg body weight (temporary).

Typical Products
Alcoholic beverages (ammonium carmine)
Foods (calcium carmine)
Red-veined cheddar
Desserts
Bakery toppings
Pie fillings
Sugar confectionery ⎰ (Ammonium carmine)
Biscuit creams
Sauces
Soft drinks

Bakery products
Drinks
Icings   } (Carmine powder)
Soups
Desserts

Now used fairly rarely because of high cost, but available as cochineal food colour for home cooking. Largely replaced by E124 in manufacturing.

E122   **Carmoisine (Azorubine; C.I. 14720)**

Source   Synthetic azo dye (see glossary).

Function   Red colour, especially for foods which are heat-treated after fermentation.

Effects   Azorubine produces no serious toxicological responses in rats, mice or pigs and does not cross the placenta in rats, but the dye is decolorized by lactic acid bacteria. The dye is broken down in the gut and eliminated in the faeces. It did not cause the genes of bacteria or a yeast to mutate. It is an azo dye, producing adverse reactions in sensitive people, or people with aspirin allergy, or asthmatics. These reactions may include urticaria (nettle rash) or oedema (water retention).

It is one of the food colours which the Hyperactive Children's Support Group recommends is eliminated from the diets of the children it represents.

A.D.I.   0–4mg/kg body weight.

Typical	Packet soup mix
Products	Blancmange
	Packet breadcrumbs
	Packet jellies
	Sweets
	Packet cheesecake mix
	Brown sauce
	Savoury convenience food mix
	Prepacked Swiss roll
	Prepacked sponge pudding
	Marzipan
	Flavoured yogurts
	Ices and ice mixes
	Jams and preserves

Its use is prohibited in Norway, Sweden, the USA and Japan.

E123 **Amaranth (C.I. 16185; FD and C Red 2)**

Source Synthetic 'coal tar' dye and azo dye (see glossary).

Function Purplish-red colour, especially useful for blackcurrant products.

Effects New studies in 1982 on metabolism and mutagenicity revealed no evidence of potential toxicity of amaranth, although the Joint FAO/WHO Expert Committee are still awaiting the results of long-term feeding studies. The dye was banned in 1976 in the United States by the Food and Drug Administration after experiments demonstrated that amaranth increased the number of malignant tumours in female rats. Some amaranth is absorbed from the food canal.

It is an azo dye, therefore to be avoided by people with aspirin sensitivity as it may cause urticaria (skin rash). This is one of the food colours which the Hyperactive Children's Support Group recommends should be excluded from the diet of the children it represents.

A.D.I.   0–0.75mg/kg body weight (temporary).

Typical   Packet soup
Products   Packet cake mix
                 Packet trifle mix
                 Liquid vitamin C preparations
                 Gravy granules
                 Tinned fruit pie fillings
                 Quick setting jelly mix
                 Ices and ice mixes
                 Jams
                 Tinned apple sauce
                 Tinned shrimps and prawns
                 Tinned pears

This colour is not permitted in Norway or the United States. In France and Italy it may only be used in caviar.

E124   **Ponceau 4R (C.I. 16255)**

Source   Synthetic 'coal tar' dye and azo dye (see glossary).

Function   Red colour.

Effects   An azo dye, so should be avoided by people with aspirin sensitivity, and by asthmatics. The colour is absorbed from the gut and excreted in the urine and faeces without tissue accumulation. Long-term studies in rats showed an absence of carcinogenic potential.

A.D.I.   0–4mg/kg body weight.

Typical	Packet trifle mix
Products	Packet cheesecake mix

Typical Products

Packet trifle mix
Packet cheesecake mix
Packet cake mix
Packet soup
Seafood dressing
Dessert topping
Tinned strawberries
Tinned cherry, redcurrant and raspberry pie
  fillings
Quick-setting jelly mix
Salami

This colour is not permitted in Norway and the
  United States.

E127 **Erythrosine (C.I. 45430; FD and C Red 3)**

Source The *di*Sodium salt of 2,4,5,7-tetraiodofluorescein, a hydrogenated derivative of fluorescein. Synthetic 'coal tar' dye (see glossary).

Function Cherry pink to red colour. Erythrosine is insoluble in acid solutions and is particularly used to colour cherries in tinned fruit cocktail as it doesn't stain the other fruit. It is also used in disclosing tablets for revealing plaque on teeth. Erythrosine is partly degraded during food processing at high temperatures over 200°C, to release iodide.

Effects Fears have been expressed that erythrosine might increase the thyroid hormone levels because of its high (577mg/gram) iodine content and lead to hyperthyroidism (overactive thyroid). Experiments were carried out with rats to see if this was so, and male rats' thyroid gland weights increased abnormally, and they developed benign tumours when they were fed diets containing 4 per cent erythrosine.

Japanese experiments show that man and rats absorb little iodine from erythrosine. The possibility still remains that large dietary intakes of erythrosine could affect the thyroid although normal intakes would not. Children consuming foods with high levels of erythrosine can have intakes approaching the levels which could cause problems.

Erythrosine has been shown to have a toxic effect on the genes of some strains of yeast cells, so the Food and Drug Administration in the United States has recommended that this dye be banned as a carcinogen. The UK Food Advisory Committee on Mutagenicity has studied the available data and advised that there is now sufficient evidence from well-conducted studies to conclude that erythrosine is probably not mutagenic.

Erythrosine has been implicated in minimal brain dysfunction in children

Erythrosine can cause phototoxicity (sensitivity to light) and when common houseflies were fed erythrosine in 0.25 and 1 per cent concentrations and were then exposed to sunlight, 100 per cent of them died within 3 hours.

A.D.I.	0–1.25mg/kg body weight. The FAC suggests a limit of 0.1mg/kg body weight.

Typical Products	Glacé cherries Cocktail cherries Tinned red cherries, strawberries and rhubarb Scotch eggs Packet trifle mix Quick custard mix

Biscuits
Prepacked Swiss roll
Stuffed olives
Chocolates
Dressed crab and salmon spread and pâtê
Garlic sausage
Luncheon meat
Danish salami

The 1987 Food Advisory Committee's recommendation is that erythrosine should be permitted in cocktail and glacé cherries only, and limited to a maximum content of 200mg/kg.

Its use is prohibited in Norway and the USA.

128	**Red 2G (C.I. 18050)**
Source	Synthetic 'coal tar' dye, and azo dye (see glossary).
Function	Red colour, particularly useful in meat products because it is not affected by sulphur dioxide (E220) and metabisulphite (E223 and E224), which bleach many colours. Not for use in foodstuffs subject to high temperature during processing, nor in products of high acidity, when red 2G hydrolyses to the amine Red 10B, a rather suspect colour.
Effects	Further toxicological studies required. The main debate on Red 2G has concerned its ability to be converted to aniline in the gut. Aniline can interfere with the haemoglobin of the red blood corpuscles, and rats fed on Red 2G have become anaemic.

It is one of the food colours which the Hyperactive Children's Support Group recommends is eliminated from the diets of the children it represents. |
| *A.D.I.* | 0–0.1mg/kg body weight. |

**Typical
Products**

Sausages
Cooked meat products
Jams
Drinks

Under consideration by the EEC for an 'E' prefix.
The 1987 Food Advisory Committee
recommendations are that Red 2G should be
restricted to meat products and vegetable
protein meat analogues, and to a maximum of
20mg/kg.

It is used in no other EEC Member State, nor is it
permitted in Switzerland, Norway, Sweden,
Finland, Austria, the United States, Canada,
Japan and Australia.

---

129   Allura Red AC (C.I. 16035; Food Red 17; FD and C Red 40)

Source

An artificial dye introduced in 1971 in the USA
to replace Amaranth (E123). An EEC draft
proposal was put forward in February 1986 but
was subsequently not approved. The FAC report
in 1987 did not oppose its use in food, but called
for further studies. Allura Red is an azo dye.

Function

Red colour.

Effects

Allura red has been shown to be non-genotoxic.
It does not cause cancer in rats or mice, but para-
cresidine, a compound used in the production
of the dye, causes bladder tumours in rodents.
No free para-cresidine has been found in food-
grade Allura Red.

There were no birth defects in rats or rabbits,
nor skin sensitivity in rabbits and man.

Of 52 people who were prone to nettle rash
or puffy skin reactions given 1 or 10mg by mouth,
8 of them responded hypersensitively.

Allura red is broken down and mostly eliminated in the faeces in the first 24 hours. The Food Advisory Committee requires further assurance that para-cresidine is not formed as a metabolite, and requested satisfactory metabolism studies within two years.

A.D.I.   0–0.7mg/kg body weight.

Typical Products   The use of Allura Red is prohibited at the time of writing in all the EEC member states. Its use is also prohibited in Austria, Norway, Sweden, Japan and Finland.

E131   Patent Blue V (C.I. 42051)

Source   Synthetic 'coal tar' dye (see glossary).

Function   Dark bluish-violet colour and diagnostic agent, used to colour the lymph vessels.

Effects   To be avoided by those with a history of allergy. Allergic reactions may occur immediately or after a few minutes. They consist of skin sensitivity, itching and urticaria (nettle rash). More severe reactions, including shock and breathing problems, occur rarely. Nausea, low blood-pressure and tremor have been reported. Detailed toxicological work has shown that Patent Blue V does not harm the genes.

It is one of the food colours which the Hyperactive Children's Support Group recommends is eliminated from the diets of the children it represents.

A.D.I.   No A.D.I. allocated.

Typical   Scotch eggs
Products

E132   **Indigo Carmine (Indigotine; C.I. 73015; FD and C Blue 2)**

Source   Synthetic 'coal tar' dye (see glossary).

Function   Blue colour and diagnostic agent (used to test whether the kidneys are functioning normally by producing blue urine after Indigo Carmine is injected into veins or muscles).

Effects   People with a history of allergy should avoid this colour. May cause nausea, vomiting, high blood-pressure and occasionally allergic reactions such as skin rash, pruritus (itching) and breathing problems.

Short-term feeding studies on dogs in the United States showed they were more sensitive to fatal viral disease when fed with this dye. Studies in Britain on the genotoxicity of this colour have proved inconclusive and further research is required.

The FAC Report on Colours 1987 makes no mention of Indigo Carmine.

It is one of the colours which the Hyperactive Children's Support Group recommends is eliminated from the diets of the children it represents.

A.D.I.   0.5mg/kg body weight.

Typical   Blancmange
Products   Biscuits
               Sweets
               Savoury convenience food mix

Its use is prohibited in Norway.

133   Brilliant Blue FCF (C.I. 42090; FD and C Blue 1)

Source   Synthetic 'coal tar' dye (see glossary).

Function   Blue colour which can produce green hues in combination with tartrazine.

Effects   This dye does not cause genes to mutate, nor is it metabolized in the food canal.

The Hyperactive Children's Support Group recommends that it should be eliminated from the diet of the children it represents.

A.D.I.   0–12.5mg/kg body weight.

Typical Products   Tinned processed peas

Under consideration by the EEC for an 'E' prefix. Its use is prohibited in Austria, Belgium, Denmark, France, Greece, Italy, Spain, Switzerland, Norway, Sweden and Germany.

E140   Chlorophyll (C.I. 75810)

Source   Chlorophyll is the green pigment in the cells of leaves responsible for absorbing light energy for photosynthesis. Pure chlorophyll is not easy to isolate and the chlorophyll which is commercially available contains other plant pigments, fatty acids and phosphatides, and is known as 'technical chlorophyll'. The usual sources are nettles, spinach, grass and lucerne. The chlorophyll is obtained by solvent extraction using acetone, ethanol, light petroleum, methyl ethyl ketone and dichloromethane. Chlorophylls may also contain other substances such as oils, fats and waxes derived from the plant material. The pigment lutein (E161(b)) may also be extracted at the same time and from the same source as chlorophyll.

Function   Olive to dark green colour. It is not a particularly stable colour and tends to fade easily.

Effects   No adverse effects are known.

A.D.I.   Not limited.

Typical
Products   Fats
                 Oils
                 Soaps
                 Naturally green vegetables and fruits preserved in a
                     liquid
                 Confectionery
                 Chewing gum
                 Ice cream
                 Soups

E141   **Copper complexes of Chlorophyll and Chlorophyllins (C.I. 75810; Copper phaeophytins)**

Source   Copper complexes of chlorophyll are derived from chlorophyll (E140) by substitution of the magnesium ion with copper, to increase stability. Copper complexes of chlorophyllins are obtained by processing of chlorophyll extracts obtained by solvent extraction from grass, spinach, lucerne, nettles and other edible plants with the addition of copper. Chlorophyllins also contain other pigments which may be presented as the copper derivative, and other substances such as the sodium or potassium salts of fatty acids, derived directly or indirectly from the source material.

Function   The copper complexes are olive-green oil-soluble colours; the chlorophyllins are green water-soluble colours.

Effects   No adverse affects are known.

A.D.I.   0–15mg/kg body weight as sum of both complexes.

Typical Products
Green vegetables and fruits preserved in a liquid
Sage Derby cheese
Parsley sauce
Ice cream
Soups
Chewing gum

E142   **Green S (Acid Brilliant Green; Food Green S; Lissamine Green; C.I. 44090)**

Source   Synthetic 'coal tar' dye (see glossary).

Function   Green colour.

Effects   Green S is poorly absorbed from the food canal except in high doses and not metabolized in rats and guinea pigs. In rats given massive doses of 1500mg/kg body weight, there was slightly increased food intake and body weight gains in males, and mild anaemia, increased protein in the urine and mild thyroid degeneration in females. None of these changes was seen at a dose of 500mg/kg.

The Food Advisory Committee had some reservations about the EEC Scientific Committee for Food's acceptable daily intake of 0–5mg/kg body weight, and suggest a figure of 0–1mg/kg body weight as being more appropriate.

A.D.I.   0–5mg/kg body weight (temporary).

Typical
Products

Packet cheesecake mix
Tinned peas
Packet breadcrumbs
Gravy granules
Mint jelly and sauce

Its use is prohibited in Norway, Sweden, Finland, Japan, Canada and the United States.

E150   Caramel colour

Source

The term 'caramel colour' relates to products of a more or less intense brown colour. It is not the sugary aromatic product obtained from heating sugar, which is used for flavouring purposes, but has poor colour intensity.

Caramel colours are dark brown to black liquids or solids having an odour of burnt sugar and a pleasant, somewhat bitter taste. They are prepared by the controlled heat treatment of carbohydrates (commercially available glucose syrup, sucrose, dextrose, invertase, etc.) in the presence of food-grade ammonia, ammonium sulphate, sulphur dioxide and/or sodium hydroxide in amounts consistent with good manufacturing practice (GMP) to promote caramelization. The number of types of caramel available has been reduced to the six proposed by the British Caramel Manufacturer's Association to meet all the needs of the British food industry.

Subsequently new specifications have been submitted by the International Technical Caramel Association, encompassing worldwide caramel products, and enabling a potential greater variability within caramels. The European Commission has proposed that the various forms of caramel be designated in the following way:

E150(a) Plain (Spirit) Caramel. Caramel prepared by the controlled heat treatment of carbohydrates with or without the presence of alkali or acids.

E150(b) Caustic Sulphite Caramel. Caramel prepared by the controlled heat treatment of carbohydrates with sulphur dioxide or sulphur containing compounds.

E150(c) Ammonia Caramel. Caramel prepared by the controlled heat treatment of carbohydrates with ammonia.

E150 Sulphite Ammonia Caramel. Caramel prepared by the controlled heat treatment of carbohydrates with ammonia and sulphite-containing caramels.

Function   Caramel colour constitutes about 98 per cent of all colouring matter added to food (approximately 8,800 tonnes/year in 1984). Depending on their method of production, the caramel colours are suitable for different products: for example, cola drinks and vinegar employ sulphite-ammonia caramel; whisky, brandy and ice cream (in the US) caustic caramel colour; and beer, stouts and gravy brownings ammonia caramel colour.

Effects   For Plain (Spirit) Caramel colour there appear to be no toxicological problems.

Industry is considering conducting short-term toxicity studies on Caustic Sulphite Caramel colour.

Because the Sulphite Ammonia Caramel colour is used so extensively in soft drinks, a lot of toxicity studies have been done on this kind of caramel colour. Rats fed high concentrations understandably find it unpalatable, drink less, eat less and lose weight. Their stools become darker coloured and soft. The caecum (first part of the large intestine) enlarges, which is thought to be associated with higher concentrations of indigestible components and is not serious, so this caramel colour is not considered to be toxic, nor does it cause reproductive abnormalities. When Sulphite Ammonia Caramel was tested on human subjects they reported gastro-intestinal symptoms including soft to liquid faeces and increased frequency of bowel movements.

Ammonia Caramel colour fed to rats decreased white cell counts, although in another experiment when rats had sufficient vitamin B_6 their white cells were not reduced. The effect of Ammonia Caramel colour on white cell count was dose-related, the lowest effect-producing dose being 200–500mg/kg body weight caramel/day. The effect was transient and reversible. The immediate health implications of this are uncertain and no experiments have taken place to discover whether other animals' white cells behave in the same way, and especially under conditions of low vitamin B_6.

Toxicological Committees seem to be seriously concerned at the difficulty in knowing which caramel colour is which, and call for greater clarity within and between the caramel colour categories which have not been chemically defined.

A.D.I.   Plain (Spirit) Caramel colour not limited.
Caustic Sulphite Caramel colour — no information.
Ammonia Caramel colour 1–100mg/kg body weight (temporary).
Sulphite Ammonia Caramel colour 0–100mg/kg body weight (temporary).

Typical Products and their Proposed A.D.I.'s

The 1987 FAC Report proposes the following upper levels for caramel colours in foods:

Non-alcoholic beverages — 1,000mg/kg
Non-alcoholic beverages to be diluted — 5,000mg/kg (before dilution)
Beer — 5,000mg/kg
Chocolate confectionery — 2,000mg/kg
Coatings and decorations for biscuits, flour confectionery, ice creams etc. — 10,000mg/kg
Crisps and similar starch-based products — 5,000mg/kg
Biscuit, bun, doughnut and pancake crumb — 5,000mg/kg
Bread, brown malt and wholemeal — 2,000mg/kg
Chocolate-flavour flour confectionery — 5,000mg/kg
Frozen desserts and dessert mixes — 5,000mg/kg
Fillings and toppings for biscuits and cakes — 5,000mg/kg
Fish and shellfish spreads and pâtés — 3,000mg/kg
Ice cream — 1,000mg/kg
Meat analogues, mycoprotein and vegetable protein — 10,000mg/kg
Milk desserts — 1,000mg/kg
Pickles, sauces, dressings and seasonings — 10,000mg/kg
Preserves — 1,000mg/kg

Sugar confectionery (sweets) including glucose
   tablets — 2,000mg/kg
Wines and spirits — limited to 5,000ml/kg

E151	**Black PN (Brilliant Black PN; C.I. 28440)**

Source   Synthetic 'coal tar' dye, and azo dye (see glossary).

Function   Black colour.

Effects   Apart from the finding of intestinal cysts in pigs given Black PN in a 90-day feeding study, no toxicologically significant effects have been observed in teratogenicity (fetal abnormality), reproduction, multigeneration, carcinogenicity or metabolic studies.

The colour is broken down by bacteria in the gut and the metabolites are readily excreted in the urine.

It is one of the colours which the Hyperactive Children's Support Group recommends is eliminated from the diets of the children it represents.

A.D.I.   0–1mg/kg body weight.

Typical   Blackcurrant cheesecake mix
Products Brown sauce
           Chocolate mousse

Its use is not permitted in Norway, Finland, Japan, Canada and the United States.

E153	**Carbon Black (Vegetable Carbon)**

Source   Carbon black can be prepared from animal charcoal, furnace black, lampblack, activated charcoal or it can be prepared in the laboratory. The main commercial source is plant material, but the source is not specified so long as the final product satisfies the purity criteria. It is unlikely that animal charcoal sources could do this.

Function   Black colour.

Effects   In 1976 Carbon Black was banned by the Food and Drugs Administration in the United States in the belief that the impurities released during dye manufacture could cause cancer.

Despite no decision having been made on an ADI, Carbon Black continues to be permitted in the EEC as specific purity criteria are said to ensure a minimum of impurities. More tests need to be done.

A.D.I.   Decision postponed.

Typical Products   Concentrated fruit juices
Jams
Jellies
Liquorice

---

154   Brown FK (Kipper Brown; Food Brown)

Source   Synthetic mixture of six azo dyes (see glossary) and subsidiary colouring matters together with sodium chloride and/or sodium sulphate as the principal uncoloured components.

Function   Brown colour, especially for kippers. In the smoking process, fish first have to be gutted and preserved by soaking in a saturated salt solution to kill bacteria, and at the same time dye (Brown FK) is added. Brown FK is considered to be the most suitable dye because it is the only colour of the correct hue stable to and soluble in brine. It produces an even colour throughout the herring flesh which does not leach or fade during storage or cooking.

A minor use is to give a 'barbecued' look to precooked poultry. Brown FK is currently permitted in all foods in the UK. The 1987 Food Advisory Committee report recommends that in future Brown FK be restricted to use in smoked and cured fish only, to a maximum level of 20mg/kg. As many people are now happy to purchase smoked fish which has not been coloured, the need for 154 must be questionable.

Effects

Experiments with bacteria have shown that two of the colour's constituents (components I and II) cause genetic mutation. When Brown FK was fed to rats and mice at huge daily oral doses (100mg/kg body weight) there was a degeneration of skeletal and heart muscle. Muscle damage also occurred after repeated oral dosing of rabbits, guinea pigs and miniature pigs. Enzyme activity was increased and disturbed and a dark pigment associated with the breakdown of enzyme bodies in the cells was apparent. The same pigment was deposited in conventional feeding studies in the rat and pig.

It is supposed that the azo dye components I and II were broken down by the gut bacteria into two amines, triamino-benzene and triameno-toluene. Both substances are mutagenic to *Salmonella* bacteria and triaminotoluene is a presumed animal carcinogen.

It is fair to assume that Brown FK is similarly metabolized in the human food canal and that potentially toxic amines will be formed, since human faeces contain gut bacteria capable of reducing these azo dyes.

The minimum concentration for Brown FK to cause gene mutation in bacteria is 1mg/1ml culture. As much as 29mg/kg dye has been found in kippers. A rough calculation is that 2 small kippers weighing 200gm each would yield enough dye for activity to be detected.

It is one of the colours which the Hyperactive Children's Support Group recommends is eliminated from the diets of the children it represents.

A.D.I. No A.D.I.

Typical Products Kippers
Smoked mackerel
Crisps
Cooked ham

Under consideration by the EEC for an 'E' prefix.
Its use is prohibited in all the EEC member states
  except the UK and the Irish Republic and in Austria, Norway, Sweden, Finland, the United States, Canada, Japan and Australia.

---

155 Brown HT (C.I. 20285; Chocolate Brown HT)

Source Synthetic 'coal tar' dye and azo dye (see glossary).

Function Brown colour, especially when manufacturers wish to use neither cocoa nor caramel in cakes.

Effects An azo dye, therefore to be avoided by people with asthma, aspirin sensitivity and skin sensitivity. It is one of the additives which the Hyperactive Children's Support Group recommends should be eliminated from the diet of the children it represents.

High oral doses of Brown HT in rats and mice led to the accumulation of a soluble pigment in the lymph nodes, but this was not found in pigs, nor long-term in rats. Brown HT undergoes azo-reduction in the food canal and is largely excreted in the urine or eliminated in the faeces in rats and guinea pigs. A small amount (0.05–0.25 per cent) has been shown to accumulate in the tissues, and some crosses the placenta. Despite this, experiments with developing animals in utero showed there were no adverse effects on survival, growth, intrauterine development, post-natal development, or on the pathology of any tissues, including the lymph nodes and kidneys. Rats given huge doses (500mg/kg) of Brown HT showed increased kidney weight and in some females caecum weight increased. (The caecum is at the junction of the large and small intestines.)

A.D.I.   0–0.25mg/kg body weight (temporary).

Typical Products   Chocolate flavour cakes

Under consideration by the EEC for an 'E' prefix.
Its use is prohibited in Austria, Belgium, Denmark, France, Norway, Sweden, Switzerland, Germany, the United States and Australia.

E160(a)   Alpha-carotene, beta-carotene, gamma-carotene (C.I. 75130)

Source   Carotenes are orange or yellow plant pigments which occur in all higher plants but are found especially in carrots, green leafy vegetables, tomatoes, apricots, rosehips and oranges. Carotenes of commerce are manufactured in the laboratory (nature-identical substances) but some commercial carotene is extracted from carrots with hexane, and consists mainly of beta-carotene, with some alpha- and gamma-carotene present. Mixed carotenes also contain other pigments and other substances such as oils, fats and waxes derived from the source material. An edible oil (e.g. peanut oil) has to be added immediately after extraction to stabilize the product.

Function Orange-yellow colour; becomes vitamin A in the body. Carotenes are insoluble in water and soluble in oils, fats and hexane. Normally stable but the colour fades on exposure to light.

Effects People with cancer have been found to have below-normal blood levels of beta-carotene and vitamin A. However, it is not yet known whether the low levels cause or result from the cancers.

A.D.I. No A.D.I.

Typical Products
Soft margarine
Butter/margarine
Yogurt dessert whip
Prepacked coffee sponge cake
Soft drinks
Milk products, condensed or dried
Foods described directly or by implication as being specially prepared for babies and young children, limited to amounts consistent with their use as vitamin sources.

E160(b) **Annatto, Bixin, Norbixin (C.I. 75120; Orlean; Rocou)**

Source A vegetable dye from the pericarp (seed coat) of the tropical Annatto tree (*Bixa orellana*). The shrub is 2 to 5 metres high. The fruit is rather like a sweet chestnut, with burrs and contains between 10 and 50 seeds covered with a thin layer of soft, slightly sticky orange pulp.

Annatto may be extracted by water-soluble or oil-soluble methods. Water-soluble annatto is extracted by agitation in aqueous alkali (sodium or potassium hydroxide) of the outer coating of the seeds. It contains Norbixin (the hydrolysis product of Bixin) as sodium or potassium salts as the major colouring principle.

Oil-soluble Annatto (as a solution or suspension) is extracted by mechanical abrasion of the outer seed coats with warm food-grade vegetable oil to separate the pericarp from the waste seeds. The major colour component is Bixin, a carotenoid.

Bixin is extracted with organic solvents such as acetone, hexane or methanol followed by removal of the solvent. The extracted Bixin may be further processed by aqueous alkali to produce Norbixin. Annatto is therefore regarded as a 'natural' colour, whereas Bixin is not.

Function   Yellow to peach or red colour, traditionally used in the dairy industry, more recently as an alternative to tartrazine. Because Annatto, Bixin and Norbixin are either oil- or water-soluble they are versatile and allow manufacturers flexibility of use. They are stable in processing and baking, and in brine which makes them useful for smoked fish.

Effects   It may not always be clear from the label which method of extraction has been used and the Hyperactive Children's Support Group reports that some people are allergic to Annatto.

There is only sparse scientific data available on Bixin.

A.D.I.	0–0.065mg/kg body weight (expressed as Bixin).

Typical Products

Margarine
Cheshire cheese
Double Gloucester cheese
Red Leicester cheese
Low-calorie spreads
Butter- or cheese-flavoured instant mashed potato
Frying oil
Carton coleslaw
Prepackaged sponge pudding
Salad cream and mayonnaise
Pastry part of steak and kidney pies
Meat balls
Fish fingers
Smoked fish
Crisps
Ice cream
Yogurts
Ice lollies
Custards
Icings
Sponge cakes
Fruit and cream fillings and toppings
Soft drinks
Liqueurs

E160(c) Capsanthin (Capsorubin; Paprika extract; Oleoresin)

Source   Paprika extract is prepared by solvent extraction of the fruit pods and seeds of *Capsicum annuum* (red pepper). Although originally a native of tropical America and cultivated by the American Indians in prehistoric times, it is the Hungarian variety (which is rather hotter than the sweet pepper used in salads) from which the paprika spice comes, but Spain is the major producer of the Capsanthin colour. The major colouring principles of paprika extracts are Capsanthin and Capsorubin, although a wide variety of other coloured compounds are present.

Function   A spice extract used primarily for its red to orange colour. Used particularly in poultry feed to deepen the colour of egg yolks. With the more widespread use of natural colours it is finding a new use in meat products.

Effects   None known. The Food Advisory Committee requested a short term oral toxicity study in rats to be submitted in 1981 but no further data have been submitted on paprika extracts.

A.D.I.   Not specified.

Typical   Processed cheese slices
Products   Egg yolks
Chicken pies

E160(d)   Lycopene (C.I. 75125)

Source   Natural plant extract from tomatoes.

Function   Red colour.

Effects   Lycopene was not considered in the Food Additives and Contaminants Committee's 1979 review of colours, and it is understood not to be currently used. Appreciable amounts of lycopene are consumed daily from sources such as tomatoes, so Lycopene was this time (1987) considered by the Food Advisory Committee to be provisionally acceptable for potential use in food, with metabolism studies required in the future.

A.D.I.	Not specified.

Typical Products	—

In contrast to the UK view there is a recent European Commission proposal that this additive be deleted.

E160(e)   beta-apo-8'-carotenal (C30; beta-8'-apocarotenal)

Source	Only synthesized pigments are available.
Function	Orange to yellowish-red colour.
Effects	No adverse effects are known.
A.D.I.	0–5mg/kg body weight as sum of the three carotenoids.

Typical Products	Cheese slices

E160(f)   Ethyl ester of beta apo-8'-carotenoic acid (C30)

Source	Only synthesized pigments are available.
Function	Natural orange to yellow colour.
Effects	No adverse effects are known.

Typical   —
Products

E161   **Xanthophylls**
E161(a)   **Flavoxanthin (C.I. 75135)**

Source   Xanthophylls are prepared by physical means and are hydroxy derivatives of alpha-, beta- and gamma-carotenes (E160a) and their naturally occurring epoxides and the fatty acid esters of those compounds present in natural food. Xanthophylls are obtained by hexane extraction of the food and subsequent removal of the solvent. The extract may then be mixed with edible vegetable oils. Xanthophylls may contain other substances, such as oils, fats and waxes derived from the source material.

Function   Yellow colour. Flavoxanthin is not commercially available.

Effects   Flavoxanthin is consumed as part of the normal daily diet and so is unlikely to pose a health hazard when used as a food colour, provided the level of use is not high.

A.D.I.   No A.D.I.

Typical   —
Products

E161   **Xanthophylls**
E161(b)   **Lutein (C.I. 75135)**

Source   Related to carotene, one of the plant pigments

present in abundance in green leaves and marigolds. Also present in egg yolks (see page 36).

Lutein is commercially available as a natural plant extract and may be obtained from the same sources and at the same time as Chlorophyll (E140).

Function Yellow to reddish colour. Used especially in poultry feed to deepen the colour of egg yolks.

Effects Lutein is consumed as part of the normal daily diet and so is unlikely to pose a hazard to health when used as a food colour, provided the level of use is not high.

A.D.I. No A.D.I.

Typical Products Eggs

The recent (1985) European Commission proposal is that this additive should be deleted.

E161 **Xanthophylls**
E161(c) **Cryptoxanthin (C.I. 75135)**

Source Related to carotene, especially well represented in the petals and berries of the *Physalis* (Bladder Cherry, Cape Gooseberry) genus (*Solanaceae*, the potato and tomato family) and also present in orange rind, egg yolk and butter.

Cryptoxanthin is not commercially available either as a plant extract or as a synthesized pigment.

Function Yellow colour.

Effects Cryptoxanthin is consumed as part of the normal daily diet and so is unlikely to pose a hazard to health when used as a food colour, provided the level of use is not high.

A.D.I.   No A.D.I.

Typical   —
Products

E161   **Xanthophylls**
E161(d)   **Rubixanthin (C.I. 75135)**

Source   Related to carotene, especially present in rosehips, but is not available commercially.

Function   Yellow colour.

Effects   Rubixanthin is consumed as part of the normal daily diet and so is unlikely to pose a health hazard when used as a food colour, provided the level of use is not high.

A.D.I.   No A.D.I.

Typical   —
Products
               The recent (1985) European Commission proposal
               is that this additive should be deleted.

E161   **Xanthophylls**
E161(e)   **Violoxanthin (C.I. 75135)**

Source   Natural extract from the plant pigment carotene, especially isolated from yellow pansies (*Viola tricolor*), but is not available commercially as a food colour.

Function	Yellow colour.
Effects	No adverse effects are known.
A.D.I.	No A.D.I.

Typical Products	The recent (1985) European Commission proposal is that this additive should be deleted.

E161   Xanthophylls
E161(f)   Rhodoxanthin (C.I. 75135)

Source	A naturally occurring carotenoid pigment found only in small amounts in, for example, the seeds of the yew tree (*Taxus baccata*). (All parts of the yew tree are poisonous, including the berries.)
Function	Yellow colour.
Effects	No adverse effects are known.
A.D.I.	No A.D.I.

Typical Products	Not commercially available. The recent (1985) European Commission proposal is that this additive should be deleted.

E161   Xanthophylls
E161(g)   Canthaxanthin (C.I. 75135)

Source	A fairly rare carotenoid pigment which can be isolated from some mushrooms, for example the chanterelle, various crustacea and fish and flamingo feathers. It can be produced

commercially as part of the synthesis of beta-carotene, or from retinal.

Function   Natural orange colour. Used on fish farms to increase the flesh pigmentation of trout and salmon, to levels at harvest of around 2–4mg/kg in trout and 8–10mg/kg in salmon, and given to flamingos in zoos to enhance the colour of their feathers.

Effects   No adverse effects are known, when canthaxanthin is taken in the amounts in which it would occur as a colour for fish, which could be 1–5mg/day, but would not be on a regular basis. Concern has been expressed because it is known from the use of canthaxanthin tablets as tanning promoters that the retina of the eye can become spotted. Users of these tablets may take 30–120mg/day for several weeks or years and have complained of deterioration of twilight-vision, sensitivity to glare and delay in dark adaptation time. As canthaxanthin is being used as a food colour increasingly because it is 'natural', in confectionery, pickles and sauces, it is thought that regular users of canthaxanthin-containing foods could be taking 1–3mg/day, and this amount is considered undesirable. The Food Advisory Committee recommend that canthaxanthin use is restricted to farmed fish and suggest that the current A.D.I. is inappropriate and should be lowered.

A.D.I.   0–25mg/kg body weight (1974) but because of the ocular problems associated with non-food use it is expected to be reduced to 0.05mg/kg body weight awaiting ophthalmological data.

Typical Products   Mallow biscuits
'Sun-tan' capsules which make the skin yellow,

simulating a tan but without sun screening
effect
Preserves, confectionery and pickles
Sauces
Trout
Salmon
Chicken pieces in breadcrumbs
Fish fingers

E162   Beetroot Red (Betanin; Betanidin)

Source   Natural extract of beetroot. The principal
colouring compound is beta-d-glucopyranoside
of betanidine.

Function   Deep purplish-red colour. Not a particularly
useful colour because of its instability in many
food-processing conditions. Also has a rather
'earthy' taste.

Effects   No adverse effects known. Beetroot Red may
contain sodium nitrate (E251) up to 25mg/kg of
the produce (in liquid or solid forms) so at high
levels there may be reasons for elimination from
the diets of babies and young children.

A.D.I.   No A.D.I.

Typical   Oxtail soup
Products   Tomato products in pizzas
Bacon burgers
Ice cream
Liquorice
Desserts
Fruit preparations
Sauces
Jams
Jellies
Sugar confectionery

E163 Anthocyanins (Schultz 1394 and 1400)

Source Anthocyanins are natural plant pigments (red, blue or violet) which are present in the cell sap of many flowers, fruits and vegetables. The most common commercially-available anthocyanin is grape-skin extract and red cabbage is another alternative. They are extracted with water, methanol or ethanol. Anthocyanins contain the common components of the source material (anthocyanin, tartaric acid, tannins, sugars, minerals, etc.).

Function Red, blue or violet food colouring. The colour obtained is pH-dependent, being reddest and most intense in very acid conditions. The shade becomes bluer as the pH rises. Anthocyanins are not suitable for the meat industry since at the pH of meat they exhibit a purple/blue colour.

Effects It seems unlikely that the consumption of anthocyanins as added food colours would significantly increase the daily intake. Information on the metabolism and toxicity of anthocyanins is limited and interpretation is complicated as there are several different, though chemically related, anthocyanins, and studies have been done with certain specific anthocyanins as well as with mixtures extracted from fruits. No adverse effects were recorded on rats or dogs fed colour from purple corn in huge amounts of 2.5g/kg and 10 per cent of the diet respectively.

Anthocyanins derived from fruits and edible plant parts are accepted by the Food Advisory Committee.

Anthocyanin extracts are permitted to contain not more than 1,000mg/kg of sulphur dioxide (E220) in liquid extracts and not more than 5,000mg/kg in dried extracts and, as sulphur dioxide is dangerous to asthmatics, anthocyanins should be avoided by this group of people.

A.D.I.   Not allocated.

Typical Products   Black cherry yogurt
Packet raspberry sorbet mix
Glacé cherries
Soft drinks
Confectionery
Tomato, carrot or vegetable soups
Jellies
Pickles
Dairy products
Ice cream

E170   Calcium carbonate (Chalk; C.I. 77220)

Source   Naturally occurring white mineral.

Function   Alkali sometimes used for deacidification of wine; firming agent for canned fruit and vegetables; releasing agent (in vitamin tablets); in calcium supplements and as a surface food colorant.

Effects   No adverse effects are known.

A.D.I.   Not specified.

Typical Products   Bread
Biscuits

Buns and cakes
Ice cream
Sweets
Vitamin and other tablets
Wine
Canned fruit and vegetables

E171   **Titanium dioxide (C.I. 77891)**

Source   Prepared from the naturally occurring mineral ilmenite.

Function   White colour to increase opacity in sauces and to provide a barrier to colour in sweets with contrasting centres.

Effects   No adverse effects are known.

A.D.I.   Not limited.

Typical   Mozzarella cheese (limited to 400mg/kg)
Products   Cottage cheese
                  Vitamin tablets and capsules
                  Horseradish cream
                  Horseradish sauce
                  Sweets
                  Lemon curd
                  Pharmaceutical tablets

                  This food colour is not permitted in Germany.

E172   **Iron oxides, iron hydroxides (yellow/brown: C.I. 77492; red: 77491; brown: 77499)**

Source   Naturally occurring pigments of iron.

Function	Yellow, red, orange, brown and black colour.

Effects The iron present in these oxides is in the ferric form and is not therefore very actively available to the body tissues. The results of feeding experiments in dogs and cats with high levels of iron did not result in any adverse effects.

A.D.I. 0–0.5mg/kg body weight.

Typical Products
Salmon and shrimp paste
Packet dessert mix
Packet cake mix
Meat paste

Use of this food colour is not permitted in Germany.

E173   Aluminium (C.I. 77000)

Source Naturally occurring, from the ore bauxite. The normal dietary intake from cereal and vegetables is 5–6mg/day.

Function Metallic colour for surface only.

Effects Insoluble forms of aluminium taken orally are poorly absorbed and of very low toxicity. Toxic effects are not seen when aluminium is present in drinking water. There is an increasing body of evidence, however, to suggest that an accumulation of aluminium in the cells of the nervous system could be potentially toxic and is found in the brain cells of people with Parkinson-type diseases and senile dementia. (Aluminium is permitted to contain not more than 10mg/kg of lead as impurities.) Several reports also suggest that a high aluminium intake may have adverse effects on the metabolism of phosphorus, calcium or fluoride in the human body and may induce or intensify skeletal abnormalities.

A.D.I.   No A.D.I.

Typical Products   Solely for external covering of dragées and the decoration of sugar-coated flour confectionery, for cake decoration and to give a silvery finish to pills and tablets.
The 1987 Food Advisory Committee recommendations placed no restriction on the maximum content of aluminium other than that of good manufacturing practice, as there is no satisfactory alternative to this colour other than silver (E174).

E174   Silver (C.I. 77820)

Source   Naturally occurring metal.

Function   Metallic surface colour.

Effects   Silver salts are toxic to bacteria and lower life-forms. Long, regular consumption can lead to argyria, a blue-grey skin, which is not dangerous. The small amounts consumed on special occasions would not accumulate in the tissues to any extent or constitute a health hazard.

A.D.I.   Decision postponed.

Typical Products   Surface colouring of chocolate confectionery, for dragées for cake decoration and sugar-coated flour confectionery.
The 1987 Food Advisory Committee

recommendations placed no restriction on the maximum silver content other than that of good manufacturing practice, as there is no satisfactory alternative to this colour other than aluminium (E173).

E175   Gold (C.I. 77480)

Source   Naturally occurring metal.

Function   Metallic surface colour.

Effects   Chemically very inactive — therefore harmless — but expensive.

A.D.I.   No A.D.I. allocated.

Typical Products   Surface colouring of chocolate confectionery dragées for cake decoration and sugar-coated flour confectionery.
The 1987 Food Advisory Committee recommendations placed no restriction on the maximum content of gold other than that of good manufacturing practice.

E180   Pigment Rubine (Lithol Rubine BK; C.I. 15850)

Source   Synthetic, an azo dye (see glossary).

Function   Reddish colour.

Effects   No adverse effects known. Toxicity studies in rats and rabbits did not show any treatment-related effects.

A.D.I.   No A.D.I. allocated.

Typical   Solely for colouring the rind of hard cheese
Products

The 1987 Food Advisory Committee recommendations placed no restriction on the use of Lithol Rubine BK on cheese rind other than that of good manufacturing practice.

E200   Sorbic acid

Source   Occurs naturally in some fruits. May be obtained from the berries of mountain ash (*Sorbus aucuparia*), and manufactured synthetically for commercial use from ketene.

Function   Preservative, inhibiting the growth of yeasts and moulds between a pH range of 4.0–6.0, but only marginally effective against bacteria. This makes sorbic acid particularly advantageous as a cheese preservative, permitting the fermenting action of lactic acid bacteria. It cannot be used in pasteurized food as it breaks down at high temperatures. Permitted in oenicological (wine-making) practices and processes.

Effects   Possible skin irritant, when directly applied. Sorbic acid is metabolized in a manner comparable with that of similar fatty acids, which is a good indication that it is unlikely to be hazardous at the current exposure level.

A.D.I.   0–25mg/kg body weight.

Typical   Fermented milks
Products   Yogurt
Gelatin capsules

Fruit salads
Sweets
Soft drinks
Bottled cheese spread
Processed cheese slices
Packet cake topping
Surface of cheese
Prepacked cake
Frozen pizza
Wine, provided that the final sorbic acid content
    does not exceed 200mg/l
Home wine kits
Candied peel
Canned cauliflower
Wine and cider
Dessert sauces
Fillings and toppings
Soup concentrates

E201   Sodium sorbate

Source   Manufactured by neutralization of sorbic acid (E200).

Function   Preservative.

Effects   None known.

A.D.I.   Not specified.

Typical Products

Frozen pizza
Margarine
Processed or non-processed cheese
Dried apricots

Foods listed under E200 (Sorbic acid) may contain sodium sorbate instead.

E202 **Potassium sorbate**

Source Manufactured by neutralization of sorbic acid (E200) with potassium hydroxide.

Function Antifungal and antibacterial preservative, more soluble than sorbic acid (E200). Permitted in oenicological (wine-making) practices and processes.

Effects None known.

A.D.I. 0–2.5mg/kg body weight.

Typical Products
Fermented milk
Yogurt
Margarine/butter spread
Cheese spread
Salad dressing
Glacé cherries
Frozen vanilla pudding
Seafood dressing
Prepacked cakes
Tinned fruit pie fillings
Frozen pizza
Preserves
Pickled cucumbers
Dried apricots
Table olives
Yogurt drink
Wine, provided that the final potassium sorbate content does not exceed 200mg/l

Foods listed under E200 (Sorbic acid) may contain Potassium sorbate instead.

E203   Calcium sorbate

Source   Manufactured by neutralization of sorbic acid (E200).

Function   Antifungal and antibacterial preservative.

Effects   None known.

A.D.I.   0–2.5mg/kg body weight.

Typical Products

Fermented milk products
Yogurt
Margarine
Concentrated pineapple juice

Foods listed under E200 (Sorbic acid) may contain Calcium sorbate instead.

E210   Benzoic acid

Source   Occurs naturally in many edible berries, fruits and vegetables. Commercially available benzoic acid is made by chemical synthesis.

Function   Preservative — antibacterial and antifungal — but effective only in an acid medium.

Effects   People who suffer from asthma or who have recurrent urticaria (nettle-rash) are likely to be sensitive to benzoic acid. It may also cause gastric irritation if consumed in large quantities. It has been reported to be responsible for neurological disorders and to react with the preservative sodium bisulphite (E222).

When hyperactive children were given a diet containing few varieties of food, and provoking foods were identified by their weekly reintroduction, benzoic acid along with tartrazine provoked a hyperactive response in 27 out of the 34 children (79 per cent). It is one of the colours which the Hyperactive Children's Support Group recommends is eliminated from the diets of the children it represents.

The body excretes benzoic acid as hippuric acid within 9–15 hours of eating food containing it.

A.D.I. 0–5mg/kg body weight.

Typical Jams
Products Beer (not exceeding 70mg/kg)
Dessert sauces
Flavouring syrups
Fruit pulp and purée
Fruit juice
Marinated herring and mackerel
Pickles
Salad cream and dressing
Fruit yogurt
Coffee essence
Margarine
Table olives
Concentrated pineapple juice
Soft drinks

Products permitted to use E210 may also use E211, E212 and E213.

E211 Sodium benzoate

Source The sodium salt of benzoic acid.

Function Preservative — antibacterial and antifungal — effective only in slightly acid environment.

Effects   People who suffer from asthma, or who have recurrent urticaria, may be sensitive to sodium benzoate and have allergic reactions. Sodium benzoate and tartrazine (E102) exacerbate the condition in between 10 and 40 per cent of patients with chronic urticaria, and possibly a higher proportion still of aspirin-sensitive individuals.

It is one of the additives which the Hyperactive Children's Support Group has added to its exclusion list.

A.D.I.   0–5mg/kg body weight.

Typical Products
Caviar
Prawns
Sweets
Margarine
Fruit pies
Soft drinks
Oyster sauce
Salad dressing
Barbecue sauce
Mexican taco sauce
Cheesecake mix
Soya sauce
Orange squash
Preserves
Pickled cucumbers
Table olives
Concentrated pineapple juice

E212   **Potassium benzoate**

Source   The potassium salt of benzoic acid.

Function   Preservative — antibacterial and antifungal.

Effects   People who suffer from asthma or are allergic to aspirin or have recurrent urticaria (nettle-rash) may be sensitive to potassium benzoate and show allergic reactions.

It is one of the additives which the Hyperactive Children's Support Group has added to its exclusion list.

A.D.I.   0–5mg/kg body weight.

Typical   Margarine
Products   Table olives
              Pickled cucumbers
              Concentrated pineapple juice

E213   **Calcium benzoate**

Source   The calcium salt of benzoic acid.

Function   Preservative — antibacterial and antifungal.

Effects   JECFA claims there are reports of a relatively high incidence of adverse reactions to calcium benzoate in susceptible individuals. They say, 'It is not clear to what extent these reactions are manifestations of immunological hypersensitivity or of idiosyncratic hyper-reactivity . . . but both can be regarded as forms of intolerance'.

People who suffer from asthma, recurrent urticaria or are allergic to aspirin are likely to be sensitive to Calcium benzoate.

It is one of the additives which the Hyperactive Children's Support Group has added to its exclusion list.

A.D.I.   0–5mg/kg body weight.

Typical Products	Concentrated pineapple juice

E214   Ethyl 4-hydroxybenzoate (Ethyl para-hydroxybenzoate)

Source   Produced from benzoic acid.

Function   Preservative — antibacterial and antifungal.

Effects   Some people are hypersensitive to benzoates, especially those sensitive to aspirin, asthmatics and those with recurrent urticaria. This substance may cause allergic contact dermatitis, although relatively few cases have been described. There is no evidence that esters of benzoic acid accumulate in the body; they are readily absorbed, broken down and excreted. There may also be a numbing effect on the mouth, as it has anaesthetic properties.

It is one of the additives which the Hyperactive Children's Support Group has added to its exclusion list.

A.D.I.   0–10mg/kg body weight.

Typical Products

Beer (not exceeding 70mg/kg)
Cooked prepacked beetroot
Chicory and coffee essence
Dessert sauces
Flavouring syrups
Flavourings
Liquid foam headings
Freeze drinks
Fruit based pie fillings
Preserved fruit — glacé, crystallized or drained
Fruit pulp or purée
Fruit juices

Marinated mackerel or herring
Salad cream
Jam

Products permitted to use E214 may also use E215.

E215 Ethyl 4-hydroxybenzoate, sodium salt (Sodium ethyl para-hydroxybenzoate)

Source   Produced from benzoic acid.

Function   Preservative — antibacterial and antifungal.

Effects   This substance may cause allergic contact dermatitis, although relatively few cases have been described. There is no evidence that esters of benzoic acid accumulate in the body; they are readily absorbed and de-esterfied. There may be a numbing effect on the mouth.

It is one of the additives which the Hyperactive Children's Support Group has added to its exclusion list.

A.D.I.   Not specified.

Typical Products   —

E216 Propyl 4-hydroxybenzoate (n-Propyl p-hydroxybenzoate; Propyl para-hydroxybenzoate)

Source   Produced from benzoic acid.

Function   Preservative — antimicrobial.

Effects   This substance may cause allergic contact dermatitis, although relatively few cases have been described. There is no evidence that esters of benzoic acid accumulate in the body; they are readily absorbed and de-esterfied. There may be a numbing effect on the mouth.

It is one of the additives which the Hyperactive Children's Support Group has added to its exclusion list.

A.D.I.   0–10mg/kg body weight.

Typical Products

Beer
Cooked prepacked beetroot
Coffee and chicory essence
Colouring matter in solution
Dessert sauces
Flavouring syrups
Freeze drinks
Fruit-based pie fillings
Fruit pulp or purée
Glucose and soft drinks
Marinated herring and mackerel
Pickles
Salad cream

Products permitted to use E216 may also use E217.

E217   **Propyl 4-hydroxybenzoate, sodium salt (Sodium n-propyl p-hydroxybenzoate; Sodium propyl para-hydroxybenzoate)**

Source   Produced from benzoic acid.

Function   Preservative — antimicrobial.

Effects   Allergic reactions to this substance may develop in asthmatics, those with recurrent urticaria (nettle-rash), or people sensitive to aspirin. There may be skin sensitivity and/or a numbing effect on the mouth.

It is one of the additives which the Hyperactive Children's Support Group has added to its exclusion list.

Propylhydroxybenzoate forms complexes in solution with methylcellulose (E461).

A.D.I.	Not specified.

Typical Products	—

E218   **Methyl 4-hydroxybenzoate (Methyl para-hydroxybenzoate; Methyl paraben)**

Source	Synthetic.
Function	Preservative — antimicrobial agent.
Effects	Some people may exhibit allergic reactions to this substance, mainly affecting the skin or mouth.

It is one of the additives which the Hyperactive Children's Support Group has added to its exclusion list. This substance is the main volatile compound in the vaginal secretions of female beagle dogs. A letter in the *Archives of Dermatology* (1985; 121: 1107) suggests that when a male dog's sexual behaviour is socially embarrassing the presence of methyl paraben may be suspected as the unwilling target of his attentions.

A.D.I.	0–10mg/kg body weight.

Typical Products	Beer (not exceeding 70mg/kg)
	Cooked prepacked beetroot
	Coffee and chicory essence
	Colouring matter in solution
	Dessert sauces
	Flavouring syrups
	Freeze drinks
	Fruit-based pie fillings
	Crystallized, glacé or drained fruit
	Glucose and soft drinks
	Marinated mackerel and herring
	Pickles
	Salad cream
	Sauces
	Snack meals
	Soup concentrates

E219

Methyl 4-hydroxybenzoate, sodium salt (Sodium methyl para-hydroxybenzoate; Sodium methyl hydroxybenzoate)

Source   Produced from benzoic acid.

Function   Preservative — active against fungi and yeasts, but less active against bacteria.

Effects   Allergic reactions have occurred when preparations containing hydroxybenzoates have been applied to the skin. Similar reactions have also occurred following intravenous or oral administration. Hydroxybenzoates have a numbing effect on the mouth.

It is one of the additives which the Hyperactive Children's Support Group has added to its exclusion list.

A.D.I.   0–10mg/kg body weight.

Typical   —
Products

E220   **Sulphur dioxide**

Source   Occurs naturally but produced chemically by the combustion of sulphur or gypsum.

Function   One of the oldest food additives known to man, Sulphur dioxide was employed by the Romans, Ancient Greeks and Egyptians as a preservative for wine. Sulphur was burnt before sealing the wine into barrels. Today it is the most reactive food additive in use and one of the most versatile, preventing food spoilage (whether it be introduced by micro-organisms, browning (enzymic or non-enzymic) or oxidation); and used as a bleaching agent for flour; as an improving agent; and for physical modification of dough in biscuit manufacture; for stabilization of vitamin C and to inhibit nitrosamine formation in the kilning of barley. It is also used in the malting process in beer-making to reduce excess loss of carbohydrate from the germinated barley rootlets, and also to prevent further growth of the barley during the dehydrating period after germination.

Seasonally available soft fruit is stored as sulphited fruit pulp to permit jam manufacture to proceed all the year round. Much of the Sulphur dioxide is lost during the jam boiling process.

It is used as a bleaching agent in the manufacture of maraschino cherries and to improve the translucency of candied citrus peels. Table grapes may be fumigated with Sulphur dioxide to inhibit *Botrytis cinerea* — a fungus which causes deterioration. Salad bars in the USA used to spray Sulphur dioxide on to salads to keep them looking fresh, excessive use causing an estimated 8 deaths from asthma.

In the wine industry Sulphur dioxide is still employed today to prevent enzymic browning in the grape must (especially important for white wines), and to inhibit the growth of lactic acid or acetic acid bacteria, ensuring the required yeast will dominate the fermentation. It stabilizes the wine colour, behaves as an antimicrobial agent and antioxidant, and traps undesirable acetaldehyde. The term 'Sulphur dioxide' as a food additive is a collective one and includes the sulphites (E221-E227).

Effects

When Sulphur dioxide dissolves, the disulphide chemical bonds which result destroy the vitamin B_1 or thiamin in foods by breaking up the protein molecules. Foods that contain a significant source of thiamine — meat, cereals, dairy products — should not be treated. This may also be the reason for sulphur dioxide's inactivation of enzymes. Bleaching of flour reduces its vitamin E content.

Sulphurous acid, produced when Sulphur dioxide is dissolved, may cause gastric irritation. Healthy people have no problem metabolizing Sulphur dioxide: the kidneys and liver both produce enzymes which oxidize sulphites, but those with impaired kidneys or liver may need to avoid sulphites.

Foods containing sulphites may precipitate an asthmatic attack in asthma sufferers, who are very sensitive to the irritant effects of sulphur dioxide gas which may be liberated from the foods containing it and inhaled as the food is swallowed.

It is one of the additives which the Hyperactive Children's Support Group recommends is eliminated from the diets of the children it represents.

A.D.I. 0–0.7mg/kg body weight.

Typical   Raspberry juice
Products Raspberry syrup
Fruit salad
Packet soup
Glacé cherries
Dried bananas and apricots
Blackcurrant jam
Desiccated coconut
Tinned cauliflower
Beer (not exceeding 70mg/kg)
Wine, cider and cider vinegar
Candied peel
Tinned crabmeat
Fruit-based milk and cream desserts
Flavourings
Freeze drinks
Fruit-based pie fillings
Crystallized, glacé or drained fruit
Fruit pulp and purée
Fruit juices
Fruit spread
Powdered garlic
Gelatin
Dry root ginger
Glucose and soft drinks
Frozen mushrooms
Dehydrated vegetables
Sausage meat

E221   Sodium sulphite

Source   A sodium salt of sulphurous acid.

Function   In food processing sulphites are used to sterilize
fermentation equipment and food containers, to

selectively inhibit undesirable micro-organisms in fermentation industries, prevent oxidative discoloration and control enzymic browning of pre-peeled and sliced/chipped apples or potatoes, especially for catering or baking use. Sulphiting agents also control non-enzymic browning. In the US sulphites were used in restaurant foods to keep salad bar vegetables and fruits looking fresh and prevent browning. Used in processing sugar beet, corn sweeteners, food starches and gelatine.

Treatment of foods with sulphites reduces their thiamine (vitamin B_1) content, so foods which contain a significant amount of thiamine — meat, cereals, dairy products — should not be treated.

In some countries sulphiting agents may be applied to specific products, e.g. fresh sausage in the UK, in which their function is to act as antimicrobial agents especially in controlling *Enterobacteriaceae* (gut bacteria) including *Salmonellae*. They also preserve the bright-red colour of meat by inhibiting the oxidation of myoglobin to metamyoglobin, and prevent the discoloration of shrimps and lobsters due to the action of the enzyme tyrosinase.

Sulphites modify the properties of dough by the sulphitolysis of disulphite bonds in the gluten. This has several technological advantages, reducing the time it takes to mix a batch of dough and reducing the elasticity of the dough. It eliminates the need for standing time for stress relaxation to occur, and allows continuous biscuit plants to make satisfactory dough sheets. They help to produce a consistent baked product even though various varieties of wheat may be used.

Effects

Asthmatics are very sensitive to the irritant effects of sulphur dioxide gas which is liberated from sulphites in acid food and inhaled when the food is swallowed. This may trigger an asthmatic attack.

In other people, ingestion of sulphites may cause gastric irritation, nausea or diarrhoea due to liberation of sulphurous acid, or allergic reactions of nettle rash or swelling (angioedema). The exact mechanism of sulphite-induced reactions is unknown.

Sulphites are oxidized by enzymes produced in the kidneys and liver; those with impaired kidneys and liver should avoid all sulphites.

The Hyperactive Children's Support Group recommends that it be avoided.

A.D.I.	0–0.7mg/kg body weight.

Typical Products	Preserved egg yolk Quick-frozen shrimps, prawns, lobsters or chips Beer, wine Concentrated pineapple juice Manufacture of caramel (E150)

E222   Sodium hydrogen sulphite (Sodium bisulphite; acid sodium sulphite)

Source	A sodium salt of sulphurous acid.
Function	Preservative for alcoholic beverages.
Effects	Since 1982 some eight deaths have been linked to the use of sulphites in the United States, a result of eating salads at salad bars which had been sprayed with sulphites in uncontrolled amounts. This practice has now been banned. All the victims had asthma. Asthmatics are very sensitive

to the irritant effects of sulphur dioxide gas which is liberated from sulphites in acid foods and inhaled as the food is swallowed. Ingestion of sulphites may cause gastric irritation in other people due to the liberation of sulphurous acid. They are a known cause of food aversion and allergic skin reactions.

Sulphites are oxidized by enzymes produced in the kidneys and liver; those with impaired organs should avoid all sulphites.

Treatment of foods with sulphites reduces their thiamine (vitamin B_1) content, so foods which contain a significant amount of thiamine, such as meat, cereals and dairy products should not be treated.

The Hyperactive Children's Support Group recommends that it be avoided.

A.D.I.	0–0.7mg/kg body weight.

Typical Products	Beer
	Wine
	Cider
	Bleaching of cod
	Bleaching of sugar
	Quick-frozen shrimps, prawns or lobsters
	Quick-frozen chips
	Dehydrated instant mashed potato
	Milk/milk products
	Fruit/juices
	Vegetables/juices
	Condiments/relish
	Gelatins/puddings/custards

E223   Sodium metabisulphite (Diosodium pyrosulphite)

Source	Commercially manufactured sodium salt of sulphurous acid.

Function   Antimicrobial preservative; anti-oxidant; bleaching agent.

Effects   Asthmatics are very sensitive to the irritant effects of sulphur dioxide gas which is liberated from Sodium metabisulphite in acid foods and inhaled as the food is swallowed. Ingestion of sulphites may cause gastric irritation in other people due to liberation of sulphurous acid.

Sulphites are known to cause food aversion and allergic skin reactions. They are oxidized by enzymes produced in the kidneys and liver; those with impaired organs should avoid all sulphites. Treatment of foods with sulphite reduces their thiamine (vitamin B_1) content, so foods which contain a significant amount of thiamine — meat, cereals, dairy products — should not be treated.

The Hyperactive Children's Support Group recommends that it be avoided.

A.D.I.   0–0.7mg/kg body weight.

Typical   Orange squash
Products   Pickled onions
             Pickled red cabbage
             Carton salad
             Packet mashed potatoes
             Quick-frozen shrimps, prawns or lobster
             Quick-frozen chips
             Sweet sauces/toppings
             Gelatins/puddings/custards
             Alcoholic beverages
             'Exotic' dried fruits and nuts

E224   Potassium metabisulphite (Potassium pyrosulphite)

Source   Commercially manufactured sodium salt of sulphurous acid.

Function	Antimicrobial preservative, especially in the Campden process for preserving fruit and home-made wine. Used to halt fermentations in breweries. Antibrowning agent.
Effects	Asthmatics are very sensitive to the irritant effects of sulphur dioxide gas which is liberated from sulphites in acid foods and inhaled as the food is swallowed. Ingestion of sulphites may cause gastric irritation due to liberation of sulphurous acid.

Effects

Asthmatics are very sensitive to the irritant effects of sulphur dioxide gas which is liberated from sulphites in acid foods and inhaled as the food is swallowed. Ingestion of sulphites may cause gastric irritation due to liberation of sulphurous acid.

Sulphites are a known cause of food aversion and allergic skin reactions. They are oxidized by enzymes produced in the liver and kidneys; those with impaired organs should avoid all sulphites. Treatment of foods with sulphites reduces their thiamine (vitamin B_1) content, so foods which contain a significant amount of thiamine — meat, cereals, dairy products — should not be treated.

The Hyperactive Children's Support Group recommends that it be avoided.

A.D.I.

0–0.7mg/kg body weight.

Typical Products

Quick-frozen chips
Quick-frozen shrimps, prawns and lobsters
Campden tablets
Wine

E226   **Calcium sulphite**

Source

A calcium salt of sulphurous acid.

Function

Preservative; firming agent in canned fruits and vegetables; disinfectant in brewing vats.

Effects   Established asthmatics are very sensitive to the irritant effects of sulphur dioxide gas which is liberated from sulphites in acid foods and inhaled in low concentrations as the food is swallowed. Ingestion of sulphite may cause gastric irritation due to the liberation of sulphurous acid.

Sulphites are a known cause of food aversion and allergic skin reactions. They are oxidized by enzymes produced in the kidney and liver; those with impaired organs should avoid all sulphites. Treatment of foods with sulphite reduces their thiamine (vitamin B_1) content, so foods containing a significant source of thiamine (meat, cereals, dairy products) should not be treated.

The Hyperactive Children's Support Group recommends that it be avoided.

A.D.I.   Not specified.

Typical Products   Cider
Fruit juices

E227   **Calcium hydrogen sulphite (Calcium bisulphite)**

Source   A calcium salt of sulphurous acid.

Function   Preservative; prevents secondary fermentation in brewing, and is used in washing beer casks to prevent the beer becoming cloudy or sour; firming agent in canned fruits and vegetables.

Effects   Established asthmatics are very sensitive to the irritant effects of sulphur dioxide gas which is liberated from sulphites in acid food and inhaled in low concentrations as the food is swallowed. Ingestion of sulphites may cause gastric irritation

131

due to liberation of sulphurous acid. Sulphites are a known cause of food aversion and allergic skin reactions. They are oxidized by enzymes produced in the kidneys and liver; those with impaired organs should avoid all sulphites. Treatment of foods with sulphite reduces their thiamine (vitamin B_1) content, and may contribute to a vitamin deficiency.

The Hyperactive Children's Support Group recommends that it be avoided.

A.D.I.	No A.D.I.

Typical Products	Beer Jams Jellies

E230   **Biphenyl (Diphenyl)**

Source   Synthetic, produced by action of heat on benzene.

Function   Fungistatic agent; food preservative which inhibits the growth of species of *Penicillium*, especially *P. digitatum*, which cause citrus fruits to go mouldy. Can penetrate the skin of fruit and might be included in food or drink prepared from fruit. Sometimes fruit is wrapped in paper impregnated with diphenyl.

Effects   More soluble in alcohol than in water, although it is considered that those consuming sufficient gin and tonic with lemon to be at risk have a substantially greater chance of cirrhosis than of harm from biphenyl. Workers exposed to diphenyl reported nausea, vomiting and irritation to eyes and nose.

A.D.I.   0–0.05mg/kg body weight.

*Typical
Products*   Treatment of skins of oranges, lemons, grapefruit
etc. Can be partly removed with detergent, but
rinse thoroughly afterwards.

Products permitted to use E230 may also use E231
and E232.

E231   2-Hydroxybiphenyl (o-Phenyl phenol; Orthophenylphenol)

Source   Prepared from phenyl ether or from dibenzo-
furan. A substance used in the manufacture of
rubber.

Function   Preservative — antibacterial and antifungal.

Effects   None known.

A.D.I.   0–0.2mg/kg body weight.

*Typical
Products*   Surfaces of citrus fruits and treatment of paper in
which they are wrapped.

Products permitted to use E231 may also use E230
and E232.

E232   Sodium biphenyl-2-yl oxide (Sodium O-phenylphenol; Sodium orthophenylphenate; Dowicide A; Natriphene)

Source   Synthetic (with a strong smell of soap).

Function   Preservative — antifungal. Alternative form of
E231.

Effects   None known.

A.D.I.   0–0.2mg/kg body weight.

Typical   Penetration of the surface of citrus fruits may
Products   cause the substance to be present in
                 marmalades and jams produced from the fruit.
             Surface of citrus fruits and paper used to wrap
                 citrus fruits.

E233   **2-(Thiazol-4-yl) benzimidazole
                (Thiabendazole; Omnizole; Thiaben;
                Tribenzole)**

Source   Prepared by the reaction of 4-thiazolecarbox-
                amide with O-phenylenediamine in polyphos-
                phoric acid.

Function   Preservative — fungicide, especially for spoilage
                control of citrus fruits. It is also used for the
                treatment of nematode worms in man.

Effects   Thiabendazole given to pregnant rats on the ninth
                day of gestation led to fetal malformations of the
                skeleton and limbs. When radioactive
                thiabendazole was fed to pregnant mice it became
                bound to large molecules in various parts of the
                body, but especially to the foetus and skeletal
                cells.

Typical   Treatment of the skins of citrus fruits and
Products   impregnating the paper in which they are
                 wrapped.
             Fresh bananas

---

234   Nisin

Source   A polypeptide antibiotic substance produced by the growth of a bacterium called *Streptococcus lactis*. Several strains of cheese starter organisms produce nisin.

Function   Preservative.

Effects   None known.

A.D.I.   33,000 units/kg body weight.

Typical   Cheese
Products   Clotted cream
               Cottage cheese
               Canned foods
               Processed cheeses

Under consideration by EEC for an 'E' prefix.

E236   Formic acid (Methanoic acid)

Source   Occurs naturally in the bodies of ants; produced commercially by heating carbon monoxide and sodium hydroxide under pressure and decomposing the resulting sodium formate with sulphuric acid.

Function   Preservative — antibacterial action; flavour adjunct.

Effects   In amounts in which it would be present in food there is no danger, although Formic acid is very caustic to the skin and if absorbed has been known to cause urine disorders. It was formerly used as a diuretic.

| A.D.I. | 0–3mg/kg body weight. |

Typical Products —

Not permitted in the UK. Member states of the EEC do not have to permit preservatives for which there is no technological need in their country.

E237 Sodium formate

Source The sodium salt manufactured from formic acid.

Function Preservative.

Effects Has diuretic properties and was formerly used for this purpose.

A.D.I. Not specified.

Typical Products —

Not permitted in the UK. See E236.

E238 Calcium formate

Source The calcium salt of formic acid.

Function Preservative.

Effects Has diuretic properties and was formerly used for this purpose.

A.D.I. Not specified.

Typical　　　—
Products

Not permitted in the UK. See E236.

E239　　　**Hexamine**
　　　　　　　(Hexamethylenetetramine)

Source　　　Manufactured from formaldehyde and ammonia.

Function　　Antimicrobial preservative.

Effects　　　Gastro-intestinal upsets may result from the prolonged use of hexamine by the production of formaldehyde. In addition, the urinary system may be affected and, less frequently, skin rashes may occur. In experiments with animals hexamine caused gene mutation and is suspected of being carcinogenic.

A.D.I.　　　0–0.15mg/kg body weight.

Typical　　　Marinated herrings and mackerel
Products　　Provolone cheese

E249　　　**Potassium nitrite**

Source　　　Potassium salt of nitrous acid.

Function　　Curing agent for meat, converting the iron-containing pigments in the flesh to stable bright-pink compounds; preservative in meat, particularly preventing the development of spores of *Clostridium botulinum*, the dangerous bacterium responsible for botulism.

Effects　　　Nitrites are capable of entering the bloodstream and changing the nature of the haemoglobin of the red blood corpuscles responsible for oxygen transport. When the blood's ability to carry oxygen is impaired there may be difficulty in breathing and pallor, dizziness or headaches, a condition known as methemoglobinemia. Infants are far more susceptible to this condition than adults, and nitrites are not permitted in foods intended for babies under six months. Nitrites are also capable of reacting with substances called amines in the stomach to form nitrosamines which are potentially carcinogenic. There is also evidence that corresponding intakes of vitamins A, C and E in the form of fresh yellow-green vegetables is protective against stomach cancer which may be why no clear relationships have been established so far between the consumption of nitrites and cancer, with the possible exception of the Icelandics.

Without the nitrates there would be many deaths from the growth of toxic micro-organisms in meats.

A.D.I. 0–0.2mg/kg body weight (temporary).

Typical Products Cooked meats
Sausages
Smoked fish

Sodium nitrite (E250) may be used instead.

E250 **Sodium nitrite**

Source Not naturally occurring; derived from sodium nitrate by chemical or bacterial action.

Function Food preservative (inhibiting the growth of

Clostridium botulinum, the bacterium responsible for botulism); curing salt, imparting a red colour to the meat.

Effects   Nitrites are capable of entering the bloodstream and changing the nature of the haemoglobin of the red blood corpuscles, responsible for oxygen transport. When the blood's ability to carry oxygen is impaired, there may be difficulty in breathing and pallor, dizziness or headaches, a condition known as methemoglobinemia. Infants are far more susceptible to this condition than adults, and nitrites are not permitted in foods intended for babies under six months.

Nitrites are also capable of reacting with substances called amines in the stomach to form nitrosamines which are potentially carcinogenic. There is also evidence that corresponding intakes of vitamins A, C and E in the form of fresh yellow-green vegetables is a considerable protection against stomach cancer which may be why no clear relationships have been established so far between the consumption of nitrites and cancer, with the possible exception of the Icelandics. A study commissioned by the US Department of Agriculture shows that 40ppm nitrite plus an inoculum of harmless bacteria (*Pediococcus acidilacti*) is as effective as the current 120ppm in preserving bacon, but results in much lower levels of nitrosamines. See E249.

It is one of the additives which the Hyperactive Children's Support Group recommends is eliminated from the diets of the children it represents.

A.D.I.   0-0.2mg/kg body weight (temporary).

Typical	Cured meat and cured meat products
Products	Salted meat, to fix the red colour
	Pork sausage
	Packet bacon steaks
	Turkey and ham loaf
	Smoked frankfurters
	Bacon
	Ham
	Tongue
	Pressed meat
	Tinned meat
	Frozen pizza
	Smoked fish

E251   Sodium nitrate (Chile saltpetre)

Source Naturally occurring mineral (especially in the Atacama desert, Chile).

Function Preservative; curing salt; colour fixative.

Effects Nitrates are capable of being converted to nitrites either when food spoils or by bacteria in the stomach (especially in tiny babies). Nitrites can cause deoxygenation of the blood or form minute amounts of nitrosamines which are hazardous poisons and potentially carcinogenic. There is also evidence that corresponding intakes of vitamins A, C and E in the form of fresh yellow-green vegetables is a considerable protection against stomach cancer (see E250).

Without the nitrates and nitrites there would be many deaths from the growth of toxic micro-organisms in meats.

It is one of the additives which the Hyperactive Children's Support Group recommends is eliminated from the diets of the children it represents.

A.D.I.   0–5mg/kg body weight.

Typical   Bacon
Products   Pressed meats
             Ham
             Tongue
             Beef
             Canned meat
             Cheese, other than Cheddar, Cheshire,
                Granapadano and Provolone
             Frozen pizza

             Potassium nitrate (E252) may be used instead.

E252   **Potassium nitrate (Saltpetre)**

Source   Naturally occurring mineral, or artificially manufactured from waste animal and vegetable material.

Function Food preservative (inhibiting the growth of *Clostridium botulinum*, the bacterium responsible for botulism); curing salt, one of the oldest and most effective ways of preserving meats; colour fixative.

Effects   Prolonged exposure to small amounts may cause anaemia, or inflammation of the kidneys. Ingestion of large quantities may cause gastroenteritis with severe abdominal pain, vomiting, vertigo, muscular weakness, and irregular pulse. Potassium nitrate may be reduced to potassium nitrite in the gut by bacterial action and this, once absorbed, can affect the haemoglobin in the red blood corpuscles preventing it carrying oxygen. Nitrites can produce minute amounts of nitrosamines which are potentially carcinogenic in man. There is also evidence that corresponding intakes of vitamins A, C and E in the form of fresh yellow-green vegetables is a considerable protection against stomach cancer (see E250). Without the nitrates and nitrites there would be many deaths from the growth of toxic micro-organisms in meats.

A.D.I.   Not specified.

Typical   Cured meats
Products   Sausages
                 Smoked frankfurters
                 Bacon, ham, tongue
                 Pressed meats
                 Tinned meats
                 Dutch cheese

E260   Acetic acid

Source   The Monsanto process uses methanol from gas or oil and carbon monoxide to manufacture acetic acid. This method is also used by BP. An older route, still used by Hoechst, produces 100 per cent acetic acid from ethanol by oxidation. It is also manufactured by the destructive distillation of wood and from acetylene and water via acetaldehyde by oxidation with air. The acetic acid in vinegar is formed by the action of the bacterium *Acetobacter* on the alcohol in beer for malt vinegar, or cider or wine for those vinegars. The sale of non-brewed condiment (i.e. 5 per cent acetic acid), as a diluted mixture is called, has been banned in France and Italy to protect the wine vinegar industry.

Function Antibacterial, and at 5 per cent concentration may be bactericidal; substance permitted to stabilize the acidity of food; diluent for colouring matter; flavouring agent; used in the malting process in beer manufacture to reduce excess losses of carbohydrate from the germinated barley rootlets, and also at the brewery acetic acid may be added to the malt slurry to compensate for variations in the water supply to produce a beer of consistent quality. Used in the bread industry to inhibit mould growth.

Effects No toxicological problems are known.

A.D.I. Not limited.

Typical Products
Foods which may provide a suitable environment for certain bacteria
Pickles
Chutneys
Cheese
Salad cream
Fruit sauce
Brown sauce
Spicy brown sauce
Mint sauce and jelly
Horseradish cream
Dilute acetic acid at about 5 per cent, called 'non-brewed condiment'
Tinned tomatoes
Tinned sardines
Tinned baby food
Edible fungi
Processed cheese preparations
Beer
Bread

E261   Potassium acetate

Source   The potassium salt of acetic acid, E260.

Function   To preserve natural colour of plant and animal tissues; buffer; neutralizing agent.

Effects   Potassium salts, taken by mouth in healthy people, cause little toxicity since potassium is rapidly excreted in the urine, but should be avoided by people with impaired kidneys.

A.D.I.   Not limited.

Typical Products   —

E262   Sodium hydrogen diacetate (Sodium diacetate; Dykon)

Source   A 'bound' compound of sodium acetate (262) and acetic acid.

Function   Acidity regulator, sequestrant, preservative — anti-microbial inhibitor especially against the spores of *Bacillus mesentericus* and *B. subtilis*. These spores are heat-resistant and, if present in bread and permitted to germinate, convert the bread into sticky yellow patches, which are capable of being pulled into long threads, hence the term 'rope'.

Effects   None known.

A.D.I.   0–15mg/kg body weight.

| *Typical* *Products* | Bread
Shaped crisps
Salt and vinegar flavour crisps |

262 Sodium acetate (anhydrous) and Sodium acetate

Source The sodium salt of acetic acid, E260.

Function Buffer (acid or alkaline stabilizer).

Effects No adverse effects are known.

A.D.I. Not limited.

| *Typical* *Products* | Bouillons
Consommés |

Under consideration by the EEC for an 'E' prefix.

E263 Calcium acetate

Source The calcium salt of acetic acid, E260.

Function Antimould agent; anti-'rope' agent (development of sticky yellow patches in bread); sequestrant; firming agent; stabilizer; buffering agent.

Effects No adverse effects are known.

A.D.I. Not limited.

| *Typical* *Products* | Packet cheesecake mix
Quick-setting jelly mix |

E270   Lactic acid

Source
Naturally occurring substance found in sour milk (as the result of the activity of lactic acid bacteria), molasses, apples and other fruit, tomato juice and in the seeds of many higher plants during germination. To produce lactic acid commercially, carbohydrates such as whey, cornstarch, potatoes or molasses are heated at high temperatures and fermented by bacteria such as *Bacillus acidilacti*, *Lactobacillus delbueckii* or *L. bulgaricus*.

Function
Food preservative; capable of increasing the antioxidant effect of other substances; acid and flavouring; used in the malting process in brewing to reduce excess losses of carbohydrate from the germinated barley rootlets. Lactic acid may be added to the malt slurry to compensate for variations in the water supply to make a beer of consistent quality.

Effects
Could cause problems in very young or premature babies who may have difficulty metabolizing it. No toxicological problems with adults.

A.D.I.
Not limited.

Typical Products
Soft margarine
Carbonated drinks
Infant milks
Confectionery
Carton salad in dressing
Salad dressing
Pickled red cabbage
Bottled cheese spread
Sauce tartare
Tinned tomatoes

Tinned pears
Tinned strawberries
Processed tomato concentrates
Jams, jellies and citrus marmalade
Tinned sardines
Tinned mackerel
Cottage cheese
Infant cereal
Tinned babyfood
Beer

E280 Propionic acid

Source A naturally occurring fatty acid, one of the products of digestion of cellulose by the gut-inhabiting bacteria of herbivorous animals. It occurs in small amounts in many foods and dairy products, acting as a natural preservative in Swiss cheese. Commercially it is obtained by one of a number of different methods: from ethylene, carbon monoxide and steam; from ethanol and carbon monoxide or by oxidation of proprion-aldehyde; from natural gas; or it can be obtained from wood pulp waste liquor by the fermentation activity of *Propionibacteria* as a by-product in the pyrolysis of wood, or in small amounts by the activity of other micro-organisms.

Function Food preservative — antifungal agent against three families of fungi.

Effects No known toxicological problems.

A.D.I. Not limited.

Typical Products Baking and dairy products
Pizza

Christmas puddings
Processed cheeses, singly or in combination with
  sorbic acid (E200) and sorbates (E201–3)

Substances permitted to use E280 may also use
  E281, E282 and E283.

E281   Sodium propionate

Source

The sodium salt of propionic acid. The propionates occur naturally in fermented foods, in human sweat and in the digestive products of ruminants.

Function

Food preservative — an antimicrobial agent against three families of moulds one of which is the 'rope' micro-organism prevalent in bread. The spores of *Bacillus mesentericus* and *B. subtilis* are heat-resistant and if present in bread and allowed to germinate, convert the bread into sticky yellow patches which can be pulled into long threads. Sodium is preferred to calcium propionate in cakes and pies.

Effects

Some reports link propionate with migraine headaches.

A.D.I.

Not limited.

Typical Products

Dairy and bakery products
Processed cheese

E282   Calcium propionate

Source

Occurs naturally in Swiss cheese; prepared commercially from propionic acid. The propionates occur naturally in fermented foods, in human sweat and in the digestive products of ruminants.

Function   Preservative — antimicrobial mould inhibitor, especially of 'rope' micro-organisms, which occur in bread. The spores of *Bacillus mesentericus* and *B. subtilis* are heat resistant and, if present in bread and permitted to germinate, convert the bread into sticky yellow patches, which are capable of being pulled into long threads.

Effects   Some reports link propionate with migraine headaches.

The Bakers' Union in the UK has banned its use in its pure form because it provokes skin rashes in bakery workers.

A.D.I.   Not limited.

Typical Products   Dairy and baking products
Frozen pizza
Processed cheese

E283   **Potassium propionate**

Source   The potassium salt of propionic acid. The propionates occur naturally in fermented foods, in human sweat and in the digestive products of ruminants.

Function   Preservative — mould inhibitor, especially of 'rope' micro-organisms which occur in bread. The spores of *Bacillus mesentericus* and *B. subtilis* are heat resistant and, if present in bread and permitted to germinate, convert the bread into sticky yellow patches, capable of being pulled into long threads.

Effects   None known.

A.D.I.   Some reports link propionates with migraine headaches.

Typical   Dairy and bakery products
Products   Christmas puddings
Processed cheese

E290   **Carbon dioxide**

Source   Natural gas, present in atmospheric air but produced by fermentation, or the action of acid on a carbonate, or as a by-product in the manufacture of lime.

Function   Preservative; coolant; freezant (liquid form); packaging gas; aerator.

Effects   Some carbonates in the stomach increase the secretion of gastric acid and promote absorption of liquid by the mucous membranes, increasing the effect of alcohol.

A.D.I.   Not specified.

Typical   Fizzy and effervescent drinks
Products   Apple juice
.   Grape juice   } preserved exclusively by
Blackcurrant juice } physical means
Cream packaged under pressure
Wine, provided that the carbon dioxide content of wine so treated does not exceed 2g/l

---

296   Malic acid (DL- or L-)

Source

Malic acid occurs in two mirror-image chemical forms, known as the D-form and the L-form. L-malic acid occurs in nature, especially in green apples, but also in pears, redcurrants, potatoes, etc., and is an important metabolite in all living cells. Commercial malic acid is usually a mixture of the D-form and the L-form and is made by chemical synthesis by heating maleic acid with dilute sulphuric acid, under pressure.

Function

Acid, flavouring.

Effects

Because it is not known whether infants can metabolize the D-form of malic acid, it is important that foods containing it are not given to babies or small children.

A.D.I.

Not specified.

Typical Products

Tinned oxtail soup
Shaped crisps
Low calorie orange squash
Packet spaghetti sauce mix
Tinned tomatoes
Tinned apple sauce
Tinned asparagus
Processed tomato concentrates
Tinned peas
Tinned strawberries
Jams, jellies and citrus marmalade
Fruit juices and nectars
Quick-frozen cauliflower
Quick-frozen sweetcorn
Quick-frozen chips

Under consideration by the EEC for an 'E' prefix.

---

297   Fumaric acid

Source   A naturally occurring organic acid especially important in cell respiration. Occurs in many plants, for example Common Fumitory (*Fumaria officinalis*), a herb used to treat eczema and dermatitis and for its laxative and diuretic properties, in the edible toadstool, *Boletus scaber* (Rough-stemmed Boletus) and in *Fomes igniarius* (a polypore fungus which grows on wood and yields a brown dye). It is prepared industrially by the fermentation of glucose by fungi such as *Rhizopus nigricans*.

Function   Acidifier and flavouring agent; raising agent and antioxidant in baked goods.

Effects   No adverse effects are known.

A.D.I.   0–6mg/kg body weight.

Typical Products   Packet cheesecake mix
Yogurt whip
Jams and jellies
Citrus marmalade

Under consideration by the EEC for an 'E' prefix.

E300   L-Ascorbic acid (Vitamin C)

Source   Naturally occurring substance in many fresh fruits and vegetables; also manufactured by biological synthesis by one of several methods. One process uses glucose which is hydrogenated to sorbitol. The bacterium, *Acetobacter suboxydans* is then employed to oxidize the sorbitol to sorbate. Further chemical additions and then heating with hydrochloric acid produces ascorbic acid. A recent single fermentation process has been achieved by transferring the genetic material of two enzymes from different bacteria to a single bacterium.

Function

Vitamin C; browning inhibitor in unprocessed cut fruits, fruit pulp and juices; improving agent for flour; meat colour preservative; used increasingly as an antioxidant in the brewing industry as more lager is produced, since the effects of oxidation are more apparent in delicately flavoured beers. Also improves shelf-life of beers, preventing haze development and 'off' flavours.

Effects

Necessary for healthy teeth, gums, bones, skin and blood vessels. Essential for growth and promotes the absorption of iron. Usually well tolerated. Large doses may cause diarrhoea and/or dental erosion. More than 10g per day could result in kidney stones in susceptible people, but this level could not be obtained from normal foods.

A.D.I.

No A.D.I. was specified for ascorbic acid when the EEC's Scientific Committee for Food completed its Review of Antioxidants in March 1986, as they felt that an A.D.I. was unnecessary in view of the low daily intake from food additive use compared with the normal daily intake from other sources (estimated as 30–100mg).

Typical Products

Concentrated fruit drinks
Tinned fruit
Fruit jams and preserves
Fruit juice
Concentrated fruit juice
Dried fruit juice
Fruit nectar

Butter
Beer
Soft and fizzy drinks
Frozen egg products
Powdered and concentrated milk
Frozen croquette potatoes
Dried potatoes (where its presence is desirable as a
     replacement for the vitamin C lost in
     processing)
Cooked and/or tinned meats
Processed cereal-based infant food
Tinned baby food
Wine, provided the final content does not exceed
     150mg/l

E301 Sodium L-ascorbate (Vitamin C; Sodium L-(+)-ascorbate)

Source   Prepared synthetically, the sodium salt of ascorbic
acid (E300).

Function   Vitamin C; antioxidant; colour preservative.

Effects   No toxicological problems in standard doses.
Some trials have shown that in rats sodium
ascorbate increases the adverse effects of known
carcinogens. The relevance of this to man needs
further research.

A.D.I.   No A.D.I. was specified for sodium ascorbate
when the EEC's Scientific Committee for Food
completed its Review of Antioxidants in March
1986, as they felt that an A.D.I. was unnecessary
in view of the low daily intake from other sources
(estimated as 30–100mg).

Typical Products

Pork pies
Scotch eggs
Sausages
Turkey and ham loaf
Smoked frankfurters
Tinned meat
Quick-frozen fish and lobster
Tinned baby food
Processed cereal-based infant food

E302 Calcium L-ascorbate (Calcium ascorbate)

Source

Prepared synthetically.

Function

Vitamin C; antioxidant; meat colour preservative.

Effects

There was some discussion in 1981 by JECFA of the theory that as oxalate is a major metabolite of ascorbate, the use of calcium ascorbate may increase the formation of calcium oxalate stones in the urine. However, they decided the intake of calcium from ascorbate in a normal diet would represent only a small fraction of the total dietary intake of calcium. It should, perhaps, be avoided by those with a predisposition to kidney stones.

A.D.I.

No A.D.I. was specified for calcium ascorbate when the EEC's Scientific Committee for Food completed its Review of Antioxidants in March 1986, as they felt that an A.D.I. was unnecessary in view of the low daily intake from food additive use compared with the normal daily intake from other sources (estimated as 30–100mg).

Typical Products	Scotch eggs
	Bouillons
	Consommés

E304 6-O-Palmitoyl-L-ascorbic acid (Ascorbyl palmitate)

Source Ascorbic acid ester produced by synthesis. Comprises ascorbic acid and palmitic acid.

Function Performs the same function as vitamin C (E300), but has the advantage at high temperatures of being fat-soluble. Antioxidant (prevents rancidity); colour preservative; prevents browning of cut fruit. An antioxidant synergistic effect exists between alpha-tocopherol (E306/7) and ascorbyl palmitate, so manufacturers are likely to use them in combination.

Effects No adverse effect known.

A.D.I. No A.D.I. was specified for ascorbyl palmitate when the EEC's Scientific Committee for Food met in March 1986, as they felt an A.D.I. was unnecessary in view of the low dietary intake from food additive use compared with the normal daily intake from other sources (estimated as 30–100mg).

Typical Products	Pork pies
	Scotch eggs
	Sausages
	Chicken stock tablets
	Infant formula
	Tinned baby food

E306   Extracts of natural origin rich in tocopherols (Vitamin E)

Source Extract of soya bean oil, wheat germ, rice germ, cottonseed, maize and green leaves, distilled in a vacuum.

Function Vitamin; antioxidant. For reasons which are not fully understood, alpha tocopherol has a greater antioxidant capacity than gamma tocopherol (E308) in animal systems, but not in cells nor in non-biological systems.

Effects Helps the supply of oxygen to the heart and muscles. It is essential for the life of the red blood cells. It acts as an antioxidant for polyunsaturated fatty acids in tissue fats and it protects other nutrients such as vitamin A from oxidation. It is largely destroyed by freezing.

A.D.I. No A.D.I. was specified for tocopherols when the EEC's Scientific Committee for Food met in March 1986, as they felt that an A.D.I. was unnecessary in view of the low daily intake from food additives compared with the normal daily intake from other sources.

Typical Products Packet dessert topping
Vegetable oils
Meat pies

E307   Synthetic alpha-tocopherol (Vitamin E; DL-alpha-tocopherol)

Source Produced by chemical synthesis.

Function Antioxidant; vitamin. It is largely destroyed by freezing.

Effects   Helps the supply of oxygen to the heart and muscles. It is essential for the life of the red blood cells. It acts as an antioxidant for polyunsaturated fatty acids in the tissue fats. It protects other nutrients such as vitamin A from oxidation.

A.D.I.   No A.D.I. was specified for tocopherols when the EEC's Scientific Committee for Food met in March 1986, as they felt that an A.D.I. was unnecessary in view of the low daily intake from food additives compared with the normal daily intake from other sources.

Typical Products   Sausages
               Pork pies

E308   **Synthetic gamma-tocopherol
                (Vitamin E; DL-gamma-tocopherol)**

Source   Produced by chemical synthesis.

Function   Antioxidant; vitamin; less effective than alpha tocopherol (E306 and E307) as a biological antioxidant (i.e. in animals), but similar capacity in a non-biological system, e.g. a polyunsaturated fatty acid or in cell cultures. It is largely destroyed by freezing.

Effects   Helps the supply of oxygen to the heart and muscles. It is essential for the life of the red blood cells. It acts as an antioxidant for polyunsaturated fatty acids in the tissue fats. It protects other nutrients such as vitamin A from oxidation.

A.D.I.   No A.D.I. was specified for tocopherols when the EEC's Scientific Committee for Food met in March 1986, as they felt that an A.D.I. was unnecessary in view of the low daily intake from food additives compared with the normal daily intake from other sources.

Typical Products	—

E309   Synthetic delta-tocopherol (Vitamin E; DL-delta-tocopherol)

Source   Produced by chemical synthesis.

Function   Antioxidant; vitamin. Delta-tocopherol is purported to be the most effective antioxidant (of all the tocopherols) in non-biological systems. It is largely destroyed by freezing.

Effects   Helps the supply of oxygen to the heart and muscles. It is essential for the life of the red blood cells. It acts as an antioxidant for polyunsaturated fatty acids in the tissue fats. It protects other nutrients such as vitamin A from oxidation.

A.D.I.   No A.D.I. was specified for tocopherols when the EEC's Scientific Committee for Food met in March 1986, as they felt that an A.D.I. was unnecessary in view of the low daily intake from food additives compared with the normal daily intake from other sources.

Typical Products   —

E310 Propyl gallate (Propyl 3,4,5, trihydroxybenzoate)

Source Propyl ester of gallic acid. Gallic acid is produced from tannins extracted from nut galls. Another method of production hydrolyses the enzyme tannase, which also occurs in spent fungal broths of *Aspergillus niger* and *Penicillium glaucum*.

Function Antioxidant in oils and fats, often in combination with BHT (E321) and BHA (E320) on which it has a synergistic (see glossary) effect.

Propyl gallate is more effective in numerous types of fats than BHA (E320), but loses much of its activity when used in baked goods, because it is unstable at high temperatures.

Effects All alkyl gallates may cause gastric or skin irritation in some people, including those who suffer from asthma or are sensitive to aspirin.

Its use is not permitted in foods intended specifically for babies or young children and it has been added to the Hyperactive Children's Support Group's exclusion list.

Propyl gallate is sometimes added to inner packaging material of foods like breakfast cereals and potato flakes, so it is possible that its vapour could contaminate the food.

A.D.I. 0–0.5mg/kg body weight for total gallates.

Typical Products Vegetable oils, margarine and shortenings singly or in combination with other gallates, or other antioxidants such as BHA (E320) or BHT (E321)
Dry breakfast cereals
Instant potato
Snack foods
Chewing gum

Chicken soup base
Potato sticks
Also used, but not declared in dairy products used
to make other foods such as butter, dried cream
or cheese, or in flavours.

E311   Octyl gallate

Source   Ester of gallic acid. Gallic acid is obtained by acid
or alkaline hydrolysis of the tannins extracted
from nut galls. Another method hydrolyses the
tannase enzyme from spent fungal broths of
Aspergillus niger and *Penicillium glaucum*.

Function   Antioxidant.

Effects   All alkyl gallates may cause gastric irritation and
problems in some people including those who
suffer from asthma or are sensitive to aspirin. Not
permitted in foods intended for babies or young
children, and it has been added to the
Hyperactive Children's Support Group's
exclusion list.

A.D.I.   0–0.5mg/kg body weight (sum of gallates).

Typical   Fats, oils and margarines, singly or in combination
Products   with other gallates.

E312   Dodecyl gallate (Dodecyl
3,4,5,-trihydroxybenzoate)

Source   Ester of gallic acid. Gallic acid is obtained by acid
or alkaline hydrolysis of the tannins extracted
from nut galls. Another method hydrolyses the
tannase enzyme from spent fungal broths of
Aspergillus niger or *Penicillium glaucum*.

Function Antioxidant.

Effects All alkyl gallates may cause gastric irritation and problems in some people including those who suffer from asthma or are sensitive to aspirin. Not permitted in foods intended for babies or young children, and it has been added to the Hyperactive Children's Support Group's exclusion list.

A.D.I. 0–0.5mg/kg body weight (sum of gallates).

Typical Products Fats, oils and margarine, singly or in combination with other gallates.

E320 **Butylated hydroxyanisole (BHA)**

Source A mixture of 2- and 3-tert-butyl-4-methoxy-phenol, prepared from p-methoxyphenol and isobutene.

Function Delays, retards or prevents the development of rancidity or other flavour deterioration in foods due to oxidation. With BHT, BHA is the most widely-used antioxidant for oils and fats either alone or with a gallate (E310-E312) and a synergist (see glossary), e.g. citric acid (E330) or phosphoric acid (E380).

It is heat resistant, so effective in baked products. Antioxidants may be lost during processing, with crisps and snack foods losing up to 90 per cent, biscuits 35 per cent. Certain commonly used cooking oils, such as soya and rapeseed, add BHA to prevent early rancidity, but others such as sunflower and safflower contain enough naturally occurring antioxidant in the form of vitamin E. It is possible that the use of added vitamin E will replace BHA and BHT in such uses. Rancidity is substantially delayed by storing oil in opaque containers.

Effects

BHA is not permitted in foods intended specifically for babies or young children, except to preserve added vitamin A.

BHA is one of the additives which the Hyperactive Children's Support Group recommends should be eliminated from the diets of the children it represents.

There is a mass of evidence to support the safety of BHA at likely levels of intake. It even seems to be a protection against some carcinogens. On the other hand there are also many scientific reports which cast doubt on its safety. At high levels there are frequent reports of toxicity, particularly its ability at high doses to promote forestomach cancers in rats and male Syrian golden hamsters. The suggestion is that BHA promotes forestomach tumours by inhibiting communication between cells, especially growth regulatory signals, and not by damaging the genes. Man does not have a forestomach so in that sense we are not at risk, but we do have similar cells lining our mouth, throat and gullet. A recent (unpublished) study by the British Industrial Biological Research Association has confirmed that BHA causes genetic changes to the ovaries of Chinese hamsters.

When BHA is used with BHT, twenty times the usual amount of BHA is stored in the body's fat. Maybe this is why undertakers report that bodies take longer to decay these days.

Increasingly, as added vitamin E or better storage and packing allow manufacturers to do without BHA, there would seem to be good reason for limiting its use. Children who eat foods containing BHA are particularly likely to consume more than the average, so their parents may be wise to choose foods free from BHA.

Some people are allergic to BHA; one study in 1977 suggested that there may be an imbalance in their body's fat metabolism.

A.D.I. 0–5mg/kg body weight (temporary). A recent study in the Netherlands estimated the daily intake of BHA to be about 4mg per person.

Typical Products

Biscuits
Sweets
Raisins
Fruit pies
Soft drinks
Margarine
Cheese spread
Sachet marinade
Beef stock cubes
Savoury rice
Packet convenience foods
Inner packaging of breakfast cereals
Vegetable oil
Shortening
Potato flakes
Crisps

BHA is not permitted for food use in Japan.

E321 **Butylated hydroxytoluene (BHT)**

Source Does not occur in nature and is prepared synthetically from p-cresol and isobutylene. It was developed initially as an antioxidant for use with petroleum and rubber products.

Function BHT delays, retards or prevents the development of rancidity and flavour deterioration in foods due to oxidation of the polyunsaturated fats and oils they contain. One of the most commonly-used antioxidants for food oils and fats, either alone, or with a gallate (E310–E312) and synergist (see glossary), e.g. citric acid (E330) or phosphoric acid (E338). BHT is much cheaper than BHA (E320) but its use in fats is limited because it is not as stable at high temperatures. Antioxidants may be lost during processing, crisps and snack foods losing up to 90 per cent, biscuits 35 per cent.

Some people are sensitive to the presence of BHT and develop rashes; they can be the same people who demonstrate aspirin sensitivity. There is a recent report in the *Lancet* of BHT causing a violent skin rash in a young French woman.

In very large doses the liver size increases, possibly because BHT is known to cause cells to divide. Even when administered in fairly low doses BHT increased the incidence of lung tumours in mice and the incidence of tumours of the liver, bladder and possibly of the food canal in rats. Yet, when rats were given BHT before a substance known to cause cancer, it (BHT) seemed to enhance the detoxification of the substance and may have protected the rats from its effects. It also acted as a chemopreventive in rat mammary tumours. Conversely it promoted bladder tumours in rats given a different substance known to cause cancer, followed by BHT. The animals given carcinogen only showed cell changes but did not develop tumours. It is claimed to be a potent inactivator of various fat-containing viruses.

When rabbits were given 1 gram of BHT per day they developed muscle weakness and died within two weeks.

Various reports have linked this additive with possible reproductive failures in experimental animals given high doses, yet rats exposed in utero to high levels of BHT produced young rats which survived better than those which had not received BHT.

It is not permitted in foods intended specifically for babies and young children. It is one of the additives which the Hyperactive Children's Support Group recommends should be eliminated from the diets of the children it represents.

A letter to the *New England Journal of Medicine* in March 1986 expressed concern that a number of university students (California University) were taking large doses of BHT for genital *Herpes simplex* virus (HSV) and for longevity. This was on the basis of advice contained in a book entitled *The Life Extension Companion*. The letter quoted the case history of the patient who took 4 grams of BHT on an empty stomach and developed cramps, weakness, nausea, vomiting, dizziness, confusion and loss of consciousness.

Increasingly, as added vitamin E, or better storage and packing is allowing manufacturers to do without BHT, there would seem to be good reason for limiting its use. Children who eat snack foods are particularly likely to consume more than the average, so their parents may be wise to choose foods free from BHT.

A.D.I.	0–0.5mg/kg body weight (temporary).

Typical Products	Margarines, shortenings and vegetable oils
	Packet cake mix
	Crisps
	Salted peanuts
	Potato rings
	Gravy granules
	Dehydrated mashed potato

Dry breakfast cereals
Chewing gum
Packet convenience foods
Inner packaging of breakfast cereals
Sachet marinade

E322   Lecithins

Source

Lecithins are mixtures or fractions of phosphatides (components of fat) obtained by physical procedures from animal or vegetable foodstuffs. Most commercial lecithin is obtained from soya beans. Other sources are egg yolk and leguminous seeds, including peanuts and maize. Lecithin is present in all living cells and is a significant constituent of nerve and brain tissues.

Function

In plant and animal cells lecithin protects the cell membranes and the polyunsaturated fats contained within the cells from oxygen attack. It is an invaluable emulsifier, lowering the surface tension of water and allowing the combination of oils and fats with water in margarine, chocolate, mayonnaise, ice cream and baked goods. Lecithin employed as an emulsifier in bread increases loaf volume, softens the crumb and extends the shelf life. In margarine it also prevents water leakage and protects vitamin A (beta-carotene). Adding a small proportion of lecithin to chocolate enables manufacturers to reduce the cocoa butter content, although the minimum is regulated. Hydroxylated lecithin is a defoaming component in yeast and beet sugar production.

Effects

Lecithin is nutritious and non-toxic. It is used

experimentally to treat senile dementia and to mobilize fats in the body.

A.D.I.   Not limited.

Typical   Chocolate
Products   Powdered milks
Soft margarine
Confectionery
Dessert mixtures
Packet trifle mix
Vermicelli
Chocolate cake covering
Yogurt whip
Chocolate biscuits
Popcorn
Bakery products

E325   **Sodium lactate**

Source   The sodium salt of lactic acid (E270).

Function   Humectant and substitute for glycerol; synergistic effect on other substances by increasing anti-oxidant effect; bodying agent.

Effects   Could have a certain toxicity because of lactose intolerance for very young children. No toxicological problems known with adults. Used medicinally as a systemic and urinary alkalizer.

A.D.I.   Not limited.

Typical   Confectionery
Products   Cheese
Jams
Jellies   } To maintain the pH level
Marmalades)

Margarine
Ice cream

E326   **Potassium lactate**

Source   The potassium salt of lactic acid (E270).

Function   Capable of increasing the antioxidant effect of other substances; buffer.

Effects   Could have a certain toxicity because of lactose intolerance for very young children. No toxicological problems known with adults. Used medicinally as a systemic and urinary alkalizer.

A.D.I.   Not limited.

Typical Products   Jams
Jellies   } To maintain the pH level
Marmalades
Ice cream

E327   **Calcium lactate**

Source   Calcium salt of lactic acid (E270). Also available commercially in hydrated forms.

Function   Antioxidant; capable of increasing antioxidant effect of other substances; buffer; firming agent; inhibits discolouration of fruits and vegetables; improves properties of dry milk powders and condensed milk; yeast food; dough conditioner.

Effects   None known. In medical use given for calcium

deficiency but may cause gastrointestinal disturbances.

A.D.I. Not limited.

Typical Products

Packet lemon meringue pie mix
Jams
Jellies ⎫
Marmalades ⎭ To maintain the pH level
Tinned tomatoes
Tinned peas
Tinned grapefruit
Tinned strawberries
Tinned tropical fruit salad

E330 **Citric acid**

Source Occurs naturally in high concentrations in lemon and other citrus juices and many ripe fruits; prepared commercially by the fermentation of molasses with fungal strains of *Aspergillus niger*. Smaller amounts are also isolated from pineapple by-products and low-grade lemons. It is available commercially in the anhydrous or monohydrate form.

Function As a synergist to enhance the effectiveness of antioxidants; prevents discolouration of fruit, development of 'off' flavours and retains vitamin C. Stabilizes the acidity of food substances; sequestrant; flavouring; helps jam to set. Used in wine production to combine with free iron to prevent the formation of iron-tannin complexes and hence cloudiness, and in the malting process in brewing to reduce excess losses of sugars from the germinated barley.

Effects   Citric acid taken in very large quantities may occasionally cause erosion of the teeth and have a local irritant action.

A.D.I.   Not limited.

Typical   Biscuits
Products   Tinned vegetables
              Tinned fruit
              Non-alcoholic drinks
              Frozen croquette potatoes
              Frozen potato waffles
              Tinned sauces
              Treatment of raisins
              Ice cream
              Packet cake mix
              Packet soup mix
              Sorbet mix
              Beer, wine and cider
              Flavouring in drinks and confectionery
              Jam, jelly and marmalade preserves
              Frozen fish, especially herrings, shrimps and crab
              Bakery products
              Cheese
              Pasteurized processed cheese
              Cheese spread
              Cream cottage cheese

Note: The highly misleading French list of dangerous additives (see page 306) states that citric acid is the most dangerous of all. This is because of the basic misunderstanding that it plays a vital role in bodily function in the Krebs cycle, and *Krebs* happens to be German for 'cancer', so citric acid therefore causes cancer! This description of the sequence of chemical reactions in virtually all cells was named after Sir Hans Krebs and has nothing to do with cancer.

E331	**Sodium citrates**
E331(a)	**Sodium dihydrogen citrate (*mono*Sodium citrate)**

Source   *Mono*Sodium salt of citric acid (E330) in the anhydrous or monohydrate form.

Function   Synergistic effect on other antioxidants; buffer to control the acidity of gelatin desserts, jams, sweets and ice cream, and retain carbonation in beverages; emulsifying salt in ice cream, processed cheese, and evaporated milk; sequestrant; added to infant milk feeds and invalid food to prevent formation of large curds. Prevents clogging of cream in aerosols and 'feathering' when cream is used in coffee.

Effects   Can alter urinary excretion of other drugs, thus making those drugs either less effective or more toxic.

A.D.I.   No A.D.I.

Typical
Products
Ice cream
Sweets
Packet Black Forest gateau mix
Processed cheese
Condensed and evaporated milks
Milk and cream powders
Marmalade
Jams
Jellies
Margarine
Ice cream

E331(b)   ***di*Sodium citrate**

Source   Sodium salt of citric acid (E330) with one-and-a-half molecules of water.

Function   Antioxidant; synergistic effect on other antioxidants; buffer; emulsifying salt.

Effects   No adverse effects are known.

A.D.I.   No available information.

*Typical
Products*   Wines
                Fizzy drinks
                Processed cheese slices

E331(c)   *tri*Sodium citrate (Citrosodine)

Source   *Tri*Sodium salt of citric acid in anhydrous, dihydrate or pentahydrate form.

Function   Antioxidant; buffer; emulsifying salt; sequestrant; stabilizer; used along with polyphosphates (E450) and flavours to inject into chickens before freezing.

Effects   No adverse effects are known.

A.D.I.   Not limited.

*Typical
Products*   Processed cheese
                Evaporated and condensed milks
                Milk powders
                Preserves
                Cooked cured meat
                Tinned baby foods
                Tinned peas
                Vegetable fats and oils
                Frozen chickens

E332   **Potassium dihydrogen citrate (*mono*Potassium citrate)**

Source   Anhydrous *mono*Potassium salt of citric acid (E330).

Function   Buffer; emulsifying salt; yeast food.

Effects   None known; potassium is rapidly excreted in the urine in healthy individuals.

A.D.I.   Not specified.

Typical Products
Sterilized and UHT cream
Condensed and evaporated milk
Dried milk
Processed cheese
Reduced-sugar jam
Fruit preserves

E332   ***tri*Potassium citrate (Potassium citrate)**

Source   A potassium salt of citric acid (E330).

Function   Antioxidant; buffer in confectionery and artificially sweetened jellies and preserves. Emulsifying salt; sequestrant.

Effects   None in foods; in therapeutic amounts when it is employed as a urinary alkalizer and gastric antacid, may make the skin sensitive and cause mouth ulcers to develop.

A.D.I.   Not limited.

Typical Products	Confectionery
	Wines
	Fizzy drinks
	Cheeses
	Rum sauce
	Crisps
	Biscuits
	Packet convenience dessert mixes and toppings
	Vegetable and animal fats and oils
	Jams
	Jellies

E333   *mono-*, *di-*, and *tri*Calcium citrate

Source Monohydrated *mono*Calcium, trihydrated *di*Calcium and tetrahydrated *tri*Calcium salts of citric acid (E330).

Function Buffers to neutralize acids in jams, jellies and confectionery; firming agents; emulsifying salts; sequestrants; improve baking properties of flour.

Effects None in foods; in therapeutic amounts may induce the formation of mouth ulcers.

A.D.I. Not limited.

Typical Products	Wines
	Fizzy drinks
	Confectionery
	Processed cheeses
	Evaporated and condensed milk
	Milk and cream powders
	Fruit preserves
	Tinned tomatoes
	Saccharine

E334   L-(+)-Tartaric acid

Source

A widely occurring fruit acid, found in grapes and other fruits either free or combined with potassium, calcium or magnesium, and sometimes deposited as crystals in wine. Tartarus is the name the medical alchemists used. Most of the L-tartaric acid is manufactured as a by-product of the wine industry (acid potassium tartrate is converted to calcium tartrate which is hydrolyzed to tartaric acid and calcium sulphate). It may also be extracted from tamarind pulp.

Function

Antioxidant; capable of increasing the antioxidant effect of other substances (synergist); to adjust acidity in frozen dairy products, jellies, bakery products, beverages, confectionery, dried egg whites, sweets, preserves and wines; sequestrant (see glossary); diluent for food colours; constituent of grape and other artificial flavours; acid in some baking powders.

Effects

Eighty per cent of the tartaric acid ingested by man is destroyed by bacteria in the intestine. The fraction absorbed into the bloodstream is excreted in the urine. Large amounts of tartaric acid have been used as a laxative without apparent harm, although strong solutions above those employed in food products are mildly irritant and may cause gastro-enteritis.

A.D.I.

0–30mg/kg body weight.

Typical Products

Confectionery
Jams
Jellies
Marmalades

Fizzy drinks
Tinned tomatoes
Tinned asparagus
Processed tomato concentrates
Tinned fruit
Cocoa powders
Frozen dairy products

E335 *mono*Sodium L-(+)-tartrate and *di*Sodium L-(+)-tartrate (Sodium L-(+)-tartrate)

Source   Monohydrated monosodium salt and dihydrated disodium salt of tartaric acid (E334).

Function   Antioxidant and capable of increasing the antioxidant effect of other substances (synergist); buffer; emulsifying salt; sequestrant.

Effects   No known toxicological risks.

A.D.I.   0–30mg/kg body weight.

Typical Products   Confectionery
Jams
Jellies
Marmalades
Fizzy drinks

E336 *mono*Potassium L-(+)-tartrate (Potassium hydrogen tartrate; Cream of tartar; Potassium acid tartrate)

Source   The Romans were probably the first to identify this substance as a fine crystalline crust during the fermentation of grape or tamarind juice. It was incorrectly termed *faecula* (little yeast) by them. It is still manufactured as a by-product of the wine industry. Anhydrous monopotassium salt of L-(+)-tartaric acid (E334).

Function	Acid; buffer especially for deacidification of wine; emulsifying salt; raising agent for flour, often used with 500 (Sodium bicarbonate) because it works slowly and gives a more prolonged evolution of carbon dioxide; inverting agent for sugar in boiled sweet manufacture.
Effects	None known; potassium salts are readily excreted by healthy kidneys. The only people at risk are those whose kidney or liver functions are impaired.
A.D.I.	0–30mg/kg body weight (as L-(+)-tartaric acid).

Typical Products	Packet lemon meringue pie mix Packet lemon meringue crunch mix Wine

E336 *di*Potassium L-(+)-tartrate

Source	*Di*Potassium salt of L-(+)-tartaric acid (E334).
Function	Antioxidant and capable of increasing the antioxidant effect of other substances (synergist); buffer; emulsifying salt.
Effects	No known toxicological risks.
A.D.I.	0–30mg/kg body weight (as L-(+)-tartaric acid).

Typical   Jelly part of packet trifle mix
Products   Packet meringue crunch mix

E337   **Potassium sodium L-(+)-tartrate (Sodium and potassium tartrate; Sodium potassium tartrate; Rochelle salt)**

Source   Derivative of L-(+)-tartaric acid (E334); available commercially in the form of potassium sodium tartrate with four molecules of water of crystallization.

Function   Buffer for confectionery and preserves; emulsifying salt; stabilizer; capable of increasing antioxidant effect of other substances (synergist).

Effects   No known toxicological problems. Used medically as a cathartic (bowel evacuation). The tartrates of the alkali metals are less readily absorbed than the citrates.

A.D.I.   0–30mg/kg body weight.

Typical   Meat and cheese products
Products   Fruit preserves
            Margarine

E338   **Orthophosphoric acid (Phosphoric acid)**

Source   There are two types of acid production, the so-called 'Wet Process' and the 'Thermal' method. 'Wet Process' involves the manufacture of phosphoric acid from phosphate ore, followed by intensive purification to meet food-grade specifications. The 'Thermal' method reduces the phosphate ore to elemental phosphorus electrothermally. Phosphorus is then burnt in air to produce phosphorus pentoxide which is dissolved in dilute phosphoric acid to create concentrated solutions. Used in concentrated aqueous solution.

Function	Capable of increasing the antioxidant effect of other substances (synergist); acidulant and flavouring agent in soft drinks, jams, frozen dairy products and sweets; used in the manufacture of cheeses which rely on the direct acidification of milk for their formation and in the brewing industry in the malting process, to reduce excess losses of sugars from the germinated barley rootlets. At the brewery, phosphoric acid may be added to the malt slurry to compensate for variations in the water supply in order to arrive at a beer of consistent quality. Sequestrant for rendered animal fat or animal and vegetable fat mixtures.
Effects	No adverse effects are known in food concentrations.
A.D.I.	0–70mg/kg body weight.

Typical Products	Fizzy drinks Cooked meats and sausages Cottage cheese Cocoa powders and dry cocoa-sugar mixtures Chocolate (as a carry-over from raw materials) Animal and vegetable fats and oils Beer

E339(a) **Sodium dihydrogen orthophosphate**
E339(b) ***di*Sodium hydrogen orthophosphate**
E339(c) ***tri*Sodium hydrogen orthophosphate**
N.B. These three chemicals are all classified as E339.

Source Prepared from phosphoric acid.

Function To improve texture and prevent seepage of serum from foods; to speed penetration of brine; antioxidant synergist; buffer; nutrient; gelling agent; stabilizer; anti-caking agent; sugar clarifying agent.

Effects High dietary intakes of phosphorus as phosphates may upset the calcium/phosphorus equilibrium.

A.D.I. 0–70mg/kg body weight.

Typical Cooked meats
Products Ham
Sausages
Processed cheese products
Instant desserts.

E340(a) **Potassium dihydrogen orthophosphate (*mono*Potassium phosphate; MKP)**
N.B. E340(a), (b) and (c) are all classified as E340.

Source Prepared from phosphoric acid.

Function Buffer; sequestrant; emulsifying salt; antioxidant synergist.

Effects Phosphorus (as phosphate) is an essential nutrient. High dietary intakes of phosphorus as phosphates, however, may upset the calcium/phosphorus equilibrium.

A.D.I.	Not specified.

Typical Products	Jelly glazing mixes Sauce mixes Instant (powdered) custard mixes Dessert topping Jelly part of packet trifle mix

E340(b)   **_di_Potassium hydrogen orthophosphate (_di_Potassium phosphate; DKP; Potassium phosphate dibasic)**

N.B. E340(b) and (c) are both classified as E340.

Source	*Di*Potassium salt of phosphoric acid (E338).
Function	Buffer; emulsifying salt; antioxidant synergist; yeast food; sequestrant.
Effects	Phosphorus (as phosphates) is essential for healthy parathyroid bone, digestive and kidney metabolism. The body can use it most efficiently if it is present in a constant ratio with calcium, so it is important that the calcium/phosphorus balance is maintained. Too much phosphorus, as phosphate, could upset the balance and cause a deficiency of both minerals. In view of the concern expressed JECFA, in 1982, recommended that further studies should be carried out on the implications of high dietary intakes of phosphorus.
A.D.I.	Not specified.

Typical Products	Non-dairy powdered coffee creamers Drinking chocolate mixes Luncheon meat

Cooked cured pork shoulder and chopped meat
Cooked cured ham
Milk and cream powders
Instant (powdered) custard mixes
Ice cream mixes

E340(c)   *tri*Potassium orthophosphate (*di*Potassium phosphate; DKP; Potassium phosphate tribasic; *tri*Potassium monophosphate)

Source   *tri*Potassium salt of phosphoric acid (E338).

Function   Emulsifying salt; antioxidant synergist; buffer; sequestrant. Phosphorus (as phosphates) is essential for healthy parathyroid, bone, digestive and kidney metabolism. This substance is not widely used in the United Kingdom.

Effects   None known.

A.D.I.   Not specified.

Typical Products   Bouillons and consommés
Luncheon meat
Cooked cured pork shoulder and chopped meat
Cooked cured ham
Instant (powdered) custard mixes
Drinking chocolate mixes

E341   Calcium orthophosphates
N.B. E341 (a), (b), (c) are all classified as E341.

E341(a) **Calcium tetrahydrogen diorthophosphate (*mono*Calcium phosphate; MCP; Acid calcium phosphate; ACP; *mono*Calcium orthophosphates; *mono*Calcium phosphate; monobasic; *mono*Basic calcium phosphate)**

Source Calcium phosphate (apatite) occurs naturally; the pulverized rock is treated with sulphuric or phosphoric acid. The food-grade product of commerce is prepared directly from high-purity phosphoric acid. *mono*Calcium phosphate is available commercially in anhydrous form or as the monohydrate.

Function Improving agent in yeast-leavened bakery products; buffer; firming agent; emulsifying salt; sequestrant; yeast food; aerator-acidulant component of self-raising flours and some baking powders; antioxidant synergist; texturizer.

Effects No adverse effects known. Phosphorus (as phosphates) is essential for healthy parathyroid, bone, digestive and kidney metabolism.

A.D.I. Not limited.

Typical Products Self-raising flour
Short pastry mix
Baking powder
Malted milk drink powder
Instant milk-based desserts
Tinned tomatoes
Cake mixes

E341(b)   **Calcium hydrogen orthophosphate (*di*Calcium phosphate; DCP; Calcium phosphate dibasic; Calcium hydrogen phosphate; Secondary calcium phosphate)**

Source   Manufactured directly from phosphoric acid.

Function   Firming agent; yeast food; nutrient mineral supplement in cereals and other foods; antioxidant synergist; animal feed supplement; abrasive in toothpaste; dough conditioner.

Effects   No adverse reactions are known, particularly as calcium phosphate is used as a calcium replenisher, dietary supplement and antacid.

A.D.I.   Not specified.

Typical Products   Tinned cherry pie filling
Milk and cream powders
Ices and ice cream mixes
Potato-based snack foods

E341(c)   **_tri_Calcium _di_orthophosphate (*tri*Calcium phosphate; Calcium phosphate tribasic)**

Source   Prepared chemically from naturally derived calcium phosphate.

Function   Anti-caking agent in icing sugar, instant (powdered) beverages, seasoning mixes and instant (powdered) soups; nutrient yeast food; diluent for vegetable extracts; clarifying agent for sugar syrups.

185

Effects	Phosphates are essential for healthy parathyroid, bone, digestive and kidney metabolism, but in balance with calcium.
A.D.I.	Not specified.

Typical Products	Cake mixes Icing sugar Powdered dextrose Evaporated and condensed milks Milk powders in vending machines Cream powders in vending machines Cocoa powders and dry cocoa-sugar mixtures (also in vending machines) Ices and ice mixes Seasoning mixes Instant (powdered) soups

350 Sodium malate

Source	A sodium salt of malic acid (296).
Function	Buffer; seasoning agent.
Effects	No adverse effects are known.
A.D.I.	Not specified.

Typical Products	Jams Jellies Citrus marmalade

Under consideration by the EEC for an 'E' prefix.

350 Sodium hydrogen malate

Source A sodium salt of malic acid (296).

Function Buffer.

Effects No adverse effects are known.

A.D.I. Not specified.

Typical Products —

Under consideration by the EEC for an 'E' prefix.

351 Potassium malate

Source The potassium salt of malic acid (296).

Function Buffer.

Effects No adverse effects are known.

A.D.I. Not specified.

Typical Products
Jams
Jellies
Citrus marmalade

Under consideration by the EEC for an 'E' prefix.

352 Calcium malate

Source A calcium salt of malic acid (296).

Function Buffer; firming agent; seasoning agent.

Effects	None known.
A.D.I.	Not specified. Included in the A.D.I. for malic acid (296) and bases.

Typical Products	Jams Jellies Citrus marmalade
	Under consideration by the EEC for an 'E' prefix.

352   Calcium hydrogen malate

Source	A calcium salt of malic acid (296).
Function	Firming agent.
Effects	No adverse effects are known.
A.D.I.	Not specified.

Typical Products	—
	Under consideration by the EEC for an 'E' prefix.

353   Metatartaric acid

Source	Prepared from tartaric acid (E334).
Function	Sequestrant, especially in wine, for precipitating excess calcium.
Effects	No adverse effects are known.
A.D.I.	Not specified.

Typical Products	Wine

Under consideration by the EEC for an 'E' prefix.

355   Adipic acid (Hexanedioic acid)

Source An organic acid which occurs in many living cells and especially in beet juice. Prepared synthetically for commercial use by oxidizing cyclohexanol with concentrated nitric acid.

Function Acidulating agent; buffer; neutralizing agent; flavouring agent for beverages and gelatin desserts to impart a smooth-tart taste; raising agent in baking powders, since, unlike tartaric acid (E334), cream of tartar (E336) and phosphates, adipic acid is not hygroscopic (water attracting).

Effects No adverse effects are known.

A.D.I. 0–5mg/kg body weight (basis on free acid).

Typical Products	Beverages Gelatin

Under consideration by the EEC for an 'E' prefix.

363   Succinic acid

Source Occurs naturally in fossils, fungi and lichens, but prepared for commercial use from acetic acid.

Function Acid; buffer; neutralizing agent.

Effects No adverse effects are known.

A.D.I.   Not specified.

Typical
Products —

Under consideration by the EEC for an 'E' prefix.

370   1,4-Heptonolactone

Source   Prepared in the laboratory: a gamma lactone made from hydroxycarboxylic acid.

Function Acid; sequestrant.

Effects   No adverse effects are known.

A.D.I.   Not specified.

Typical
Products —

Under consideration by the EEC for an 'E' prefix.

375   Nicotinic acid (Niacin; Nicotinamide)

Source   Occurs naturally in yeast, liver, legumes, rice polishings and lean meats, although it is prepared for commercial use by the oxidation of nicotine with concentrated nitric acid.

Function B vitamin; colour protector.

Effects   Nutrient essential for the conversion of food into energy, and aiding the maintenance of a normal nervous system. Nicotinic acid can dilate the blood vessels and, if given in therapeutic doses, it may produce flushing of the face, and pounding in the head and a sensation of heat. It is perfectly safe in normal food use.

A.D.I.   Not specified.

Typical   Bread
Products   Flour
               Breakfast cereals

               Under consideration by the EEC for an 'E' prefix.

380   *tri*Ammonium citrate (Citric acid *tri*Ammonium salt; Ammonium citrate tribasic)

Source   The salt of citric acid (E330), which dissolves easily in water, releasing free acid.

Function   Buffer; emulsifying salt to blend pasteurized processed cheese and cheese foods; softening agent for cheese spreads.

Effects   Citrates may interfere with the results of laboratory tests, including tests for pancreatic function, abnormal liver function and blood alkalinity-acidity.

A.D.I.   Not specified.

Typical   Processed cheeses
Products   Cheese spreads

               Under consideration by the EEC for an 'E' prefix.

381   Ammonium ferric citrate (Ferric ammonium citrate)

Source	Prepared from citric acid (E330).
Function	Dietary iron supplement; used medically for raising the level of red blood cells.
Effects	Iron is an essential mineral nutrient, preventing anaemia.
A.D.I.	Not specified.

Typical Products	Iron tablets Infant milk formulae Bread flour (not 100 per cent wholemeal)
	Under consideration by the EEC for an 'E' prefix.

381   Ammonium ferric citrate, green

Source	Prepared from citric acid.
Function	Dietary iron supplement.
Effects	Iron is an essential mineral nutrient, preventing anaemia.
A.D.I.	Not specified.

Typical Products	—
	Under consideration by the EEC for an 'E' prefix.

385 **Calcium disodium ethylenediamine-NNN'N' tetra-acetate (Calcium disodium EDTA; Edetate)**

Source Prepared synthetically.

Function Traces of free metal ions of aluminium, copper, zinc, iron, manganese or nickel are likely to occur in any manufactured food which has come into contact with machinery. Positively charged, these ions are likely to combine with substances in the food to spoil it by discolouration, cloudiness, rancidity or unpleasant smells. EDTA acts as a 'chelating agent', attracting the positively charged ions by trapping them in its own negatively charged ones and rendering them inactive. EDTA is soluble in water but not in oil, so it can only be used in water-based foods or oil-water mixtures. In some senses it functions as an antioxidant.

Effects Intravenous injections of EDTA are a long-established moderately successful treatment for lead poisoning, but oral administration of large amounts of EDTA in excess of that normally used in foods has caused vomiting, diarrhoea, abdominal cramps, kidney damage and blood in urine. It is important that the manufacturer adds only enough EDTA to bind the metal impurities *in the food*, as excess EDTA could combine with the body's essential metallic elements such as iron, zinc and copper, and prevent their utilization.

A.D.I. 0–2.5mg/kg body weight.

Typical Products *UK permitted use only in*:
Canned fish and shellfish

Glacé cherries

Under consideration by the EEC for an 'E' prefix. Member States were allowed to authorize the use of calcium disodium EDTA until the end of 1986.

E400   **Alginic acid**

Source   Extracted from brown seaweeds, the most widely used being species of *Laminaria* (British Isles, France, Norway, North America, Japan), *Macrocystis* (USA) and *Ascophyllum* (British Isles).

The alginate (or algin as it is sometimes called) is present in seaweed as a mixed sodium, potassium, calcium and magnesium salt of alginic acid. The seaweed is dried and then macerated and broken down with a dilute alkaline solution to extract the alginate. The alginate is precipitated from solution as the insoluble calcium salt, and further treated and purified to produce alginic acid — from which all the other alginates (E401-E405) are made. The basic extraction method has changed little since alginate was first isolated in about 1880. Commercial utilization in the food industry began in 1934.

Function   Alginic acid is insoluble in cold water and is therefore rarely used as a food additive.

Effects   This is a natural product which produces no known toxicological risks. In common with other soluble fibres, very large quantities, greater than those likely in any normal diet, can inhibit the absorption of certain nutrients, especially minerals and trace elements.

A.D.I.   0–50mg/kg body weight.

Typical   Ice lollies
Products   Suspending agent in soft drinks
             Puddings
             Instant desserts
             Custard tarts, etc.
             Jams
             Spray cream
             Yogurt
             Bakery glaze

E401   Sodium alginate

Source   Extracted from brown seaweeds, especially
             Laminaria, and produced as part of the
             manufacture of alginic acid (E400) of which it is
             the sodium salt.

Function   Stabilizer, suspending agent and thickening agent.
             Also used, in combination with a source of
             calcium, as a gelling agent. Copper (i.e. the
             container in which the wort is boiled) fining agent
             in brewing to encourage the precipitation and
             coagulation of proteins and tannins.

Effects   This is a natural product which produces no
             known toxicological risks. In common with other
             soluble fibres, very large quantities, greater than
             those likely in any normal diet, can inhibit the
             absorption of certain nutrients, especially
             minerals and trace elements.

A.D.I.   0–50mg/kg body weight.

Typical *Products*	*Stabilizer:* Ice cream Ice lollies Soft cheese Imitation cream Yogurt Low-sugar jams *Suspending agent:* Fruit drinks *Thickening agent:* Sauces Syrups *Gelling agent:* Instant desserts Jellies and puddings Potato croquettes Onion rings Stuffed olives Fruit pie fillings Baker's custard *Copper firming agent:* Beer

---

E402   Potassium alginate (Potassium polymannuronate)

Source   Prepared from alginic acid (E400) derived from native brown seaweeds. The potassium salt of alginic acid (E400).

Function   Emulsifier; stabilizer; boiled water additive; gelling agent.

Effects   This is a natural product which produces no known toxicological risks. In common with other soluble fibres, very large quantities, greater than those likely in any normal diet, can inhibit the absorption of certain nutrients, especially mineral and trace elements.

196

A.D.I.	0–25mg/kg body weight (calculated as alginic acid (E400).

Typical Products	Although a permitted additive, it is rarely (if ever) used as such in foodstuffs, sodium alginate (E401), which has similar properties, being preferred. May be used in diets when the sodium level is being controlled.

E403   **Ammonium alginate**

Source	Prepared from alginic acid (E400) derived from native seaweeds. It is the ammonium salt of alginic acid (E400).

Function	Emulsifier; stabilizer; diluent for colouring matter; thickener.

Effects	This is a natural product which produces no known toxicological risks. In common with other soluble fibres, very large quantities, greater than those likely in any normal diet, can inhibit the absorption of certain nutrients, especially mineral and trace elements.

A.D.I.	0–50mg/kg body weight.

Typical Products	Icings

E404   **Calcium alginate (Algin)**

Source	Prepared from alginic acid (E400) derived from

native brown seaweeds. The calcium salt of alginic acid.

Function   The addition of calcium to algin solutions produces gels which are very stable, so calcium alginate is a useful emulsifier, stabilizer, thickener and gelling agent. It is also added to jam to prevent it oozing out of oven-baked pastry foods.

Effects   This is a naturally derived product which produces no known toxicological risks. In common with other soluble fibres, very large quantities, greater than those likely in any normal diet, can inhibit the absorption of certain nutrients, especially minerals and trace elements.

A.D.I.   0–25mg/kg body weight (as alginic acid (E400)).

Typical Products
Ice cream
Synthetic cream
Tinned green beans and peas
Tinned sweetcorn
Tinned mushrooms
Tinned asparagus
Tinned carrots
Processed cheese preparations
Cottage cheese
Cream cheese
Tinned sardines
Pickled cucumbers
Whipped pasteurized cream
UHT cream
Sterilized cream for whipping
Flavoured yogurt
Ice lollies

E405 **Propane-1,2-diol alginate
(Propylene glycol alginate;
alginate ester)**

Source The propylene glycol ester of alginic acid (E400) derived from native brown seaweeds. It varies in composition according to its degree of esterification and the percentage of free and neutralized carboxyl groups in the molecule.

Function Emulsifier or stabilizer, especially in ice cream, water ices and salad dressings; thickener; solvent for extracts, flavours or spices; foam stabilizing agent (helps to maintain a stable 'head' on light lagers and ales to compensate for loss of hops and malts or degradation of proteins by proteolytic enzymes added to prevent haze formation).

Effects None known. The Food Additives and Contaminants Committee who prepared the Report on the Review of Additives and Processing Aids used in the Production of Beer in 1978 stated that, if toxicological information on E405 was not available by 1980, it would not be prepared to recommend its continued use.

A.D.I. 0–25mg/kg body weight.

---

*Typical
Products*
Thousand Island dressing
Cottage cheese with salmon and cucumber
Mint sauce
Seafood dressing
Carton salad
Orange squash
Light lagers and ales
Tinned vegetables
Processed cheese preparations
Cream cheese

Ice lollies
Beer, provided the level does not exceed 100mg/l

E406   Agar (agar-agar; Japanese isinglass)

Source

'Agar-agar' is a Malay word and describes the mucilage produced from a red seaweed. In the last century, Japan was the only exporter of agar, but it has now been joined by Spain and Portugal, New Zealand, Korea, South Africa and the USA. *Gelidium amansii* was the original seaweed used to produce agar; other members of the Gelidiaceae family are also used today and members of the Sphaerococcaceae and related red algae Rhodophyceae. The algae are dried and bleached on the shore and then pounded, washed and boiled. The extract is filtered through linen, cooled and frozen to remove water, and dried. It is sold in strips or powder form. Not to be confused with isinglass which is the swim bladders of fish.

Function

A colloidal carbohydrate, agar produces rather firm, brittle gels which are not as effective in foods as carrageenan (E407) or gelatin. It is used as a thickening agent, stabilizer and gelling agent, and as a humectant for icings on cakes. It is also used as a copper (i.e. the container in which the beer wort is boiled) firming agent in brewing to encourage the precipitation and coagulation of proteins and tannins.

Effects

Agar is not digested; large quantities of it may temporarily increase flatulence and distension or cause intestinal obstruction, but it is likely that amounts in food are too small to produce these effects. In common with other soluble fibres, very large quantities, greater than those likely in any normal diet, can inhibit the absorption of certain nutrients, especially minerals and trace elements. It is used medically as a bulk laxative.

A.D.I.   Not limited.

Typical   Thickening agent for ice cream and for glazing
Products   meats when a firm jelly is needed
Frozen raspberry trifle
Beverages
Meringue
Baked goods
Icings
Confectionery
Artificially sweetened jams and preserves
Milk
Cream
Flavoured yogurt
Ice lollies
Tinned cod's roe

E407   Carrageenan

Source   'Irish moss' is another name for carrageenan and the Irish have used a seaweed extract in milk puddings, food and medicine for some 600 years. It was not produced commercially, however, until the Second World War when an alternative to (Japanese) agar (E406) was sought. Until the 1950s it was mainly extracted on a commercial scale in the USA, but expanding demand extended industrial production to Scandinavia and France.

It occurs in about 22 species of red seaweeds belonging to the Gigartinaceae, Solieriaceae, Hypnaceae and Furcellariaceae families and is recovered commercially from *Chondrus* seaweed in the United States and *Chondrus crispus* and *Gigartina sp.* in Europe.

The seaweeds are dried mechanically or are left on the shore to be alternately bleached and soaked, and then dried. They are then washed to remove salts and debris before the extraction process using alkaline hot water. The resulting dried mucilage is translucent and swells in cold water, partially dissolving to produce a jelly. The extract is concentrated to about 3 per cent carrageenan before alcohol is added to precipitate it.

'Carrageenan' describes a number of complex hydrocolloids rather than a single substance. It consists of varying amounts (depending on the processing methods) of the ammonium, calcium, magnesium, potassium or sodium salts of sulphate esters of galactose and 3,6-anhydro-galactose copolymers. The sulphate ester content of carrageenan ranges from 18–40 per cent. The principal copolymers are designated *kappa-*, *lambda-* and *iota-* and these three copolymers differ in structure and in their gelling ability. They are termed 'native' carrageenan, or 'undegraded' carrageenan, meaning that the long polysaccharide molecules of carrageenan have not been sub-divided or split. The carrageenan used in food has a high molecular weight (1 to 8,000,000). 'Degraded' carrageenan has a very low molecular weight (20–30,000) and no gelling properties.

Food-grade carrageenan *must* comprise the long-chain molecules and must not be degraded.

Function Stabilizing, thickening, suspending and gelling agent. It imparts the desired body and texture to foods, especially dairy products. It is used in concentrations of 0.01–1.0 per cent. It also has many uses in the fields of drugs and cosmetics as well as having wider industrial applications.

Effects Some confusion has arisen because *degraded* carrageenan (the kind which is *not* permitted in food use) has induced ulcerative colitis in a wide range of laboratory animals, and tumours of the colon and rectum. To ensure that degraded carrageenan is never used in food, the current EEC statutory specification for purity requires that 'carrageenan shall not be hydrolysed or otherwise be chemically degraded' and seeks to ensure this by imposing a minimum viscosity requirement on a solution of the material treated under standardized conditions. A study commissioned by MAFF and 'written up in a form not suitable for publication' said all the (21) samples investigated met the statutory requirement and of those few (4) subjected to molecular weight fractionation, in all cases low molecular weight material accounted for only 5 per cent of the total polysaccharide present (personal communication, John Howlett, Food Science Division, MAFF).

The complex polysaccharide may be degraded a little in the acid environment of the stomach, but not enough to cause any harm. The question of whether more degradation occurs during rigorous food processing conditions of acid pH and high temperatures has not been satisfactorily resolved.

Native (undegraded) carrageenan on its own and administered in the diets of laboratory animals did not cause tumours to develop. When it was fed to rats with azomethane or N-nitrosomethylurea, all the rats fed carrageenan *plus one of these substances* developed colon tumours, whereas only *some* of the controls fed *no carrageenan but one or other of the substances* developed tumours.

When six patients with malignant colon disease were given 5g degraded carrageenan daily for ten days before having a colectomy, there were no signs of any ulceration nor of absorption of the carrageenan. No pathological effects were seen in rhesus monkeys fed 500mg/kg a day for seven and a half years, but they had soft stools and diarrhoea.

Guinea pigs, rabbits and mice showed changes in the mucous membranes of the caecum, colon and rectum resembling those found in ulcerative colitis in man when they were fed concentrations of undegraded carrageenan ranging from 0.1 per cent to 1 per cent in the drinking water.

It was therefore surprising that when the Joint Expert Committee on Food Additives in 1984 reviewed the A.D.I. for carrageenan which had previously been 75mg/kg body weight, they allocated it the most favourable standing of 'A.D.I. not specified'. This evaluation means that the total daily intake of carrageenan, arising from its use at the levels necessary to achieve the desired effect and from its acceptable background in food, does not represent a hazard to health. We believe that until further relevant trials prove otherwise the intake of large regular amounts of carrageenan has not been shown to be totally safe.

A.D.I.	Not specified.

Typical Products	Evaporated and condensed milks Chocolate milk Milk-based beverages, e.g. alcoholic milk drink, egg nog UHT sterilized cream Low calorie spreads Milk shakes, especially thick milk shakes

Blancmange, pudding and custard mixes
Instant mousse mixes
Quick-setting jelly mixes
Ice cream mixes
Ice cream
Water ices
Yogurt
Buttermilk
Sour cream
Reformed fruit and vegetable pieces
Artificial glacé cherries
Structured pimento strips for olive stuffing
Re-formed meat pieces
Artificially sweetened jam
Textured sausages
Pork pies
Re-formed fish pieces
Jellified anchovy paste for stuffing olives
Biscuits
Pastries
Tinned pet foods
Soya milk
Toothpaste

E410   Locust bean gum
(Ceratonia gum, Carob bean gum)

Source   The Locust or Carob tree (*Ceratonia siliqua*) is an evergreen tree belonging to the Leguminoseae or pea family native to the Mediterranean region. It produces pods which bear shiny brown seeds and it is the endosperm or stored food in the seeds which constitutes the carob bean gum. Carob powder (the chocolate substitute) is manufactured from the pod of the same plant. Carob bean gum was used by the ancient Egyptians for mummy binding and the sugary pods, rich in protein, have been eaten since biblical times (St John's Bread). They are used for stock feed today. Locust bean gum is a high molecular weight polysaccharide composed of galactopyranose and mannopyranose units and known as galactomannan.

Function   Gelling agent; stabilizer for ice creams; emulsifier; thickening agent for soups, salad dressings and pie fillings; texture modifier in cheeses, cake and biscuit doughs. It helps to make carrageenan (E407) gels softer and more palatable.

Effects   None known. Two American reports, one from the University of Minnesota, suggest that locust bean gum may lower blood cholesterol levels. In common with other soluble fibres very large quantities, greater than those likely in any normal diet, can inhibit the absorption of certain nutrients, especially minerals and trace elements.

A.D.I.   A temporary A.D.I. 'Not specified'. was allocated in the 19th JECFA Report and this was extended in the 24th Report (1980). The Committee reviewed the considerable body of available toxicological data and removed the temporary status of the A.D.I.

Typical Products
Jelly part of packet trifle mix
Italian ice cream
Tinned cherry pie filling
Carton salad (celery, apple and orange)
Salad cream
Aerosol cream
Syrups for frozen products
Confectionery
Cream cheese
Water ices
Tinned vegetables
Tinned fish
Flavoured yogurts

E412 Guar gum (Jaguar gum, Guar flour, Cluster bean)

Source A gum extracted from the stored food in the seeds of *Cyamopsis tetragonolobus*, or *C. psoraloides*, a member of the pea family native to India and the drier topics and grown in the south-western areas of the United States as a cattle feed.

Function Thickening agent; emulsion stabilizer; suspending agent; dietary bulking agent; helps diabetics control blood sugar levels.

Effects Adverse effects only occur when excessively large quantities are consumed and can include nausea, flatulence and abdominal cramps. In common with other soluble fibres, very large quantities, greater than those likely in any normal diet, can inhibit the absorption of certain nutrients, especially minerals and trace elements. A positive effect is the reported reduction in blood cholesterol levels.

A.D.I. Not specified.

Typical Products
Bottled barbecue sauce
Carton salad
Scotch eggs
Salad dressings
Packet soups
Packet meringue crunch mix
Tinned chicken in white sauce
Brown sauce
Piccalilli
Horseradish cream
Sauce tartare
Carton coleslaw
Milk shake
Ice cream

Frozen fruit
Icings and glazes
Fruit drinks
Cream cheese
Yogurt

E413   **Tragacanth**
              (Gum dragon, Gum tragacanth)

Source   Tragacanth gum exudes from the trunk and
              branches of *Astragalus gummifer* and other
              species of the same genera (pea family). It may
              flow naturally, but is more usually collected by
              incision — as rubber is — from small thorny
              bushes which grow sparsely in mountain
              locations in Iran, Iraq, Turkey, Russia and other
              parts of the Middle East. The exudate is a ribbon
              of soft tragacanth, varying in colour and quality
              according to the age of the bushes and the degree
              of burning received by the tops of the bushes.
              White or pale-yellow gum is used in pharmacy,
              while the amber, reddish or brown flakes are used
              in the food and textile industries. Powdered
              tragacanth is pale-yellow or white in colour.
              Chemically it consists mainly of high molecular
              weight polysaccharides composed of galacto-
              arabans and acidic polysaccharides containing
              galacturonic acid groups.

Function   Emulsifier; stabilizer; thickener (especially in
              acidic foods); prevention of crystallization in sugar
              confectionery; used in cake decorating in the
              home to convert royal icing to a paste which can
              be moulded with the fingers.

Effects   Adverse reactions have only occurred rarely and
              contact dermatitis has been reported when

tragacanth was used on the skin. Tragacanth has been used as an emulsifier since pre-Christian times and can be ingested in large amounts with impunity, although diarrhoea, flatulence or constipation may result.

When five healthy male volunteers consumed 9.9g gum tragacanth daily for twenty-one days there were no adverse toxicological effects. The intestine transit time and the fat content of the stools increased in four of the men, but all the other parameters measured (blood cholesterol, urine analysis, glucose tolerance, etc.) were normal.

A.D.I.   No A.D.I.

Typical
Products   Cottage cheese with salmon and cucumber
Cake decorations
Piccalilli
Salad dressings
Processed cheese
Cream cheese
Fruit sherberts
Fruit jam
Water ices
Sweets
Flavoured yogurt

E414   **Gum arabic (Acacia; Sudan gum; Gum hashab; Kordofan gum)**

Source   The dried gum which flows from the stems and branches of *Acacia senegal* and related species (members of the pea family). It collects and dries in walnut-sized globules. After an incision has been made in the bark, the dried tears or globules are collected and exported without further processing apart from the removal of foreign objects. The most important region for gum arabic production is Kordofan in the Sudan, but the gum-yielding acacia trees grow along a 3,000km wide band following the southern frontier of the Sahara desert from West Africa to the Middle East, and in India.

The Egyptians used acacia gum more than 4,000 years ago as an ingredient in paints. Chemically, it consists of high molecular weight polysaccharides mainly with their calcium, potassium and magnesium salts, which on hydrolysis yield arabinose, galactose, rhamnose and glucuronic acid.

Function

To retard sugar crystallization; thickener of sweets, jellies, glazes and chewing gum and to convert royal icing into a plastic paste in home cake decorating; emulsifier; stabilizer preventing chemical breakdown in food mixtures and maintaining the foam on beer and soft drinks; glazing agent; and used to help citrus and other oily flavours to be added to drinks. Gum arabic is the most readily water-soluble of all the vegetable gums. It is also used as a copper (i.e. the container in which the wort is boiled) firming agent in brewing to encourage the precipitation and coagulation of proteins and tannins.

Effects

A few people have demonstrated hypersensitivity to gum arabic after breathing it in or eating it, but it is used medically as a demulcent to soothe irritations, especially of the mucous membranes, and has been shown to lower the cholesterol levels in the blood of rats.

When five healthy men ate 25g gum arabic daily for twenty-one days there was no effect on glucose tolerance, stool weight or appearance.

There was a slight reduction in cholesterol in the blood. It seems that gum arabic is largely degraded in the human colon.

The extensive data available from studies in animals and in man and the detailed chemical data available suggest gum arabic is one of the most extensively evaluated food additives. No upper level limits were specified by the FAO/WHO Committee, reflecting its safety as a food additive.

A.D.I.   Not specified.

Typical   Fruit gums
Products   Packet Black Forest gateau mix
             Tinned vegetables
             Wine
             Beer

E415   **Xanthan gum (Corn sugar gum)**

Source   Produced by the fermentation of a carbohydrate such as corn sugar with a bacterium called *Xanthomonas campestris* in the presence of nitrogen and mineral nutrients.

Function Stabilizer, thickener, and emulsifier for water-based foods such as dairy products and salad dressings. It can form a thick gel on standing, but is quite liquid when shaken, stirred or poured, so is a useful 'pseudoplasticizer' in salad dressings, helping them to pour well. Used in cake mixes to improve appearance and to allow fewer eggs or less water to be used without affecting the result. When xanthan gum and guar gum (E412) are present together in the ratio 2:1 (xanthan to guar) gelation is enhanced.

Effects   The low A.D.I. allocated to xanthan gum

compared with other gums does not imply that E415 is less desirable, but reflects the problems associated with administering very viscous hydrocolloids to small laboratory animals. No adverse effects attributable to xanthan gum have been reported in toxicological tests on rodents. When five male volunteers consumed xanthan gum in weights equal to fifteen times the current A.D.I., on each of twenty-three consecutive days their faecal weight increased, as did faecal transit time. Their blood and urine analyses remained the same and there was a moderate reduction in serum cholesterol, with an increase in faecal bile acids.

A.D.I.　　　0–10mg/kg body weight.

Typical 　　Seafood dressings
Products　　Carton coleslaw and carton salads
　　　　　　 Horseradish cream
　　　　　　 Frozen pizza
　　　　　　 Packet dessert topping
　　　　　　 Tinned cherry pie filling
　　　　　　 Sweet pickle
　　　　　　 Packet cake mix
　　　　　　 Tinned sponge pudding

416　Karaya gum (Sterculia gum; Indian tragacanth)

Source　　An exudate from the trunk and stems of the tree *Sterculia urens* native to central India and Pakistan. The trees are tapped and the gum harvested twice a year. It collects in irregular-shaped masses which can weigh up to several pounds each and varies in colour and quality depending on the amount of impurities contained. The top grades are colourless and translucent.

Function Stabilizer; emulsifier; thickener; prevents ice-crystals from forming in ice cream and binds fat and juices to meat in sausages. Used as a filler in lemon custard and as citrus and spice flavouring agent for beverages, ice creams and sweets. Karaya gum can attract and absorb sufficient water to multiply its original volume one hundred times.

Effects A few people are allergic to karaya gum which indicates that some of it is absorbed. It can function as a laxative, so little of it is digested, but it is not known how the presence of the substance in the gut affects the absorption of nutrients.

When five healthy male volunteers consumed 10.5g of Karaya gum (a very large amount in relation to the amount in foods) daily there was no toxic effect on intestinal transit time, faecal weight or composition, glucose tolerance, serum cholesterol or any other of the parameters measured. Karaya gum had no metabolic action of any consequence.

A.D.I. 0–20mg/kg body weight (temporary).

Typical Products
Some cheeses
Fruit sauce
Spicy brown sauce
Piccalilli
Ices
Ice cream
Sweets
Baked goods
Beverages
Under consideration by the EEC for an 'E' prefix.

E420(i) **Sorbitol**
E420(ii) **Sorbitol syrup**

Source A six-carbon sugar alcohol which was first discovered in the ripe fruits of Mountain ash (*Sorbus aucuparia*). It occurs in the fruits of other members of the same family (Rosaceae), notably in cherries, pears, plums and apples and also in seaweeds and other algae. It is metabolized in the body. Commercial sources are from glucose by high-pressure hydrogenation or electrolytic reduction. Sorbitol syrup is an aqueous solution of sorbitol and hydrogenated oligosaccharides.

Function Sweetening agent and substitute for glycerol. When added to syrups containing sucrose it reduces the tendency to deposit crystals on storage extending the product's shelf-life. Sorbitol masks the bitter after-taste of saccharin in drinks and helps to maintain the physical texture of chewy sweets. Also used as a humectant, stabilizer and texturizer.

Effects Sorbitol is converted to sugar in the bloodstream, but it is only absorbed slowly, making it a useful source of sugar for diabetics, and reducing the incidence of dental caries. The Food Standards Committee in 1976 considered Sorbitol to be an undesirable ingredient for general use in soft drinks since some people have a low gastric tolerance for Sorbitol. It was recommended that its use in soft drinks be limited to those intended for consumption by diabetics. Large amounts (30g for children, 60g for adults) could cause flatulence, abdominal distension or have a laxative effect, but it is well-tolerated. Sorbitol is not permitted in foods intended specifically for babies or young children.

A.D.I.	Not specified.

Typical Products	Chocolates Confectionery Pastries Ice cream Food colour diluent Diabetic jam Prepackaged cakes Raisins

E421 Mannitol (Manna sugar)

Source Occurs naturally in the wood of coniferous trees. Generally prepared from seaweed or manna, the dried exudate of *Fraxinus ornus* (Manna ash) which grows in Sicily and the 'toe' of Italy. The French tamarisk (*Tamarix gallica var. mannifera*) which grows on the south coast produces a similar exudate to seal the bark when it has been attacked by scale insects. The biblical manna which fed the Israelites may have been the wind-blown dispersal of a lichen called *Lecanora esculenta* native to the Middle East and used by Arabs to produce a bread. Strong winds can tear it from its substrate and transport it considerable distances. Commercial mannitol is usually prepared by hydrogenation of invert sugar (glucose and fructose), monosaccharides and sucrose.

Function Texturizing agent; dietary supplement; humectant; sweetener in sugar-free products; anti-caking agent; anti-sticking agent.

Effects Mannitol has been used for centuries as a sweetener with no adverse effects. About two-

A POSITIVE REACTION TO PRESSURES

The ingredients lists below are taken from two identical examples of a popular snack product, both with the same front labels and both bought in the same supermarket on the same day.

The first example had a 'sell by' date of February 1987, and the second a 'sell by' date of April 1987.

Compare the lists of ingredients.

Sell by February 1987

Ingredients. Wheatflour, Vegetable Oil with Antioxidants (E320, E321), Cheese & Tomato Flavour (Flavour Enhancer (621), Flavouring, Colours (E102, E110, E124, 154, Acidity Regulators (E262, E331), Acetic Acid, Citric Acid, Artificial Sweetener (Saccharin), Maltodextrin, Salt, Tomato, Sweetcorn, Chives, Preservative (E220).
Sachet: Tomato Sauce.

Sell by April 1987

Ingredients: Wheatflour, Vegetable Oil, Cheese & Tomato Flavour (Flavourings, Flavour Enhancers (621, 635), Artificial Sweetener (Saccharin), Maltodextrin, Salt, Tomato, Sweetcorn, Chives, Colour (Annatto), Preservative (E220).
Sachet: Tomato Sauce.

thirds of it is absorbed in the digestive tract of which some is excreted in the urine. Of the total intake only about half is assimilated, which reduces the relative calorific value of food sweetened with mannitol compared with sugar. It also reduces the incidence of dental caries. Hypersensitivity reactions have occurred occasionally and mannitol may cause nausea, vomiting and diarrhoea. It may also induce or exacerbate kidney disease. Not permitted in foods intended specifically for babies or young children.

A.D.I. —

Typical Products
Sweets
Ice cream
Chewing gum

E422 **Glycerol (Glycerin)**

Source
Occurs naturally in many plant cells, synthesized by the plants themselves. It is an industrial by-product in the manufacture of soaps, candles and fatty acids from oils and fats. With the decline in the demand for soap and increasing use of detergents, other methods had to be found. Alternative methods synthesize glycerol from propylene or by fermentation from sugars.

Function
Solvent for oily chemicals, particularly flavourings which are soluble in water; humectant (keeping foods moist) in marshmallows, pastilles and jelly-sweets; sweetener (about 0.6 times as sweet as cane sugar); bodying agent in combination with

gelatins and edible gums; plasticizer in edible coatings for meat and cheese.

Effects   Glycerol is a common substance in the body's biochemistry, as an energy source and as a component of more complex molecules. It is readily absorbed from the intestine and metabolized to carbon dioxide and glycogen (animal starch) or used in the synthesis of body fats. 'Binge' eating can produce effects such as headache, thirst, nausea and high blood sugar levels. It is mildly laxative.

A.D.I.   Not specified.

Typical Products
Liqueurs
Confectionery
Cake icing
Coatings for meat and cheese
Beverages
Baked goods
Chewing gum
Gelatin desserts
Marshmallows
Fudge

---

430   Polyoxyethylene (8) stearate (Polyoxyl 8 stearate)

Source   A mixture of stearate and ethylene oxide.

Function   Emulsifier; stabilizer.

Effects   Some people who have allergic skin reactions are allergic to macrogol stearate. There has been some suggestion that this additive may have an effect on the gastrointestinal and urinary tracts, forming kidney stones etc.

A.D.I.   0–25mg/kg body weight.

Typical Products   Bakery foods

Under consideration by the EEC for an 'E' prefix.

431   Polyoxyethylene (40) stearate (Polyoxyl 40 stearate)

Source   A waxy solid which is a mixture of stearate and ethylene oxide.

Function   Emulsifier; added to bread to make it 'feel fresh'.

Effects   When this substance was fed to undernourished rats deficient in vitamin A it produced a proliferation of stomach cells and hence was a cancer hazard, although well-nourished rats showed no such reaction.

A.D.I.   0–25mg/kg body weight.

Typical Products   Bread

Under consideration by the EEC for an 'E' prefix.

432   Polyoxyethylene (20) sorbitan monolaurate (Polysorbate 20; Tween 20)

Source   A complex mixture of partial lauric esters of sorbitol and its mono- and di-anhydrides condensed with ethylene oxide.

Function   Emulsifier; stabilizer; dispersing agent. It is more hydrophilic (water-attracting) than Polysorbate 60 (435) and Polysorbate 80 (433).

Effects   Polysorbate emulsifiers have been in use since the 1940s and because of their efficiency are only necessary in concentrations of 0.01 per cent. They may increase the absorption of liquid paraffin and other fat-soluble substances and have sometimes been used clinically to treat those with deficient fat absorption.

A.D.I.   0–25mg/kg body weight.

Typical Products   —

The use of the polysorbates has been extended until 31.12.88, during which time these substances must be re-evaluated by the Commission.

433   Polyoxyethylene (20) sorbitan mono-oleate (Polysorbate 80; Tween 80)

Source   A complex mixture of partial oleic esters of sorbitol and sorbitol anhydride copolymerized with ethylene oxide.

Function   Emulsifier and defoamer in the production of sugar beet; stabilizer; keeps bread rolls and doughnuts moist; prevents oil leaking from artificial whipped cream; helps the solubility of non-dairy coffee whiteners.

Effects   Polysorbate emulsifiers have been in use since the 1940s and, because of their efficiency, are only necessary in concentrations of 0.01 per cent. They may increase the absorption of liquid paraffin and other fat-soluble substances.

A.D.I.   0–25mg/kg body weight.

Typical   Chocolate mousse
Products   Artificial cream
              Bakery products
              Non-dairy coffee whiteners
              Sweets
              Ice cream
              Beverages

The use of the polysorbates has been extended until 31.12.88, during which time these substances must be re-evaluated by the Commission.

434   Polyoxyethylene (20) sorbitan monopalmitate (Polysorbate 40; Tween 40)

Source   A palmitate ester of sorbitol and sorbitol anhydride copolymerized with ethylene oxide.

Function   Emulsifier; stabilizer; dispersing agent (especially of flavours); defoaming agent; wetting agent for powdered processed foods.

Effects   Polysorbate emulsifiers have been in use since the 1940s and because of their efficiency are only necessary in concentrations of 0.01 per cent. They may increase the absorption of liquid paraffin and other fat-soluble substances.

A.D.I.   0–25mg/kg body weight.

Typical
Products

Cakes and cake mixes
Whipped mixes
Whipped vegetable oil toppings
Cake icings and fillings
Ice cream
Frozen desserts
Non-dairy coffee whiteners

The use of the polysorbates has been extended until 31.12.88, during which time these substances must be re-evaluated by the Commission.

435   Polyoxyethylene (20) sorbitan monostearate (Polysorbate 60; Tween 60)

Source

A complex mixture of partial stearic acid esters of sorbitol and its mono- and di-anhydrides condensed with ethylene oxide.

Function

Emulsifier; stabilizer — especially in frozen desserts to prevent the oil and water separating out and creating wetness; prevents oil leaking from artificial whipped cream and flavour oils leaking from sweets; keeps bread and doughnuts moist; wetting and dispersing agent for powdered processed foods like non-dairy coffe whiteners; added to chocolate coatings to prevent the fat used as a substitute for cocoa fat from tasting greasy; foaming agent in non-alcoholic beverage mix to be added to alcoholic beverages.

Effects

Polysorbates may increase the absorption of liquid paraffin and other fat-soluble substances. The American Food and Drug Administration has asked for further studies of this additive.

A.D.I.   0–25mg/kg body weight.

Typical   Packet cake mix
Products   Bread
                Doughnuts
                Non-dairy coffee whiteners
                Chocolate coatings
                Non-alcoholic beverage mix
                Whipped vegetable oil topping
                Cakes and cake mixes
                Cake icings and fillings
                Sugar-type confectionery coatings
                Confectionery
                Chicken bases
                Gelatin desserts
                Dressings made without egg yolks

                Under consideration by the EEC for an 'E' prefix.

436   Polyoxyethylene (20) sorbitan tristearate (Polysorbate 65; Tween 65)

Source   A stearic acid ester of sorbitol and sorbitol anhydride copolymerized with ethylene oxide.

Function   Emulsifier, especially in frozen desserts, preventing the oil and water from separating out and producing wetness; prevents oil leaking out of artificial whipped cream and flavour oils leaking from sweets; stabilizer; keeps bread and doughnuts moist; wetting and solution agent for processed dehydrated foods like non-dairy coffee whiteners; defoaming agent; flavour dispersing agent.

Effects   Polysorbate emulsifiers have been in use since the 1940s and because of their efficiency are only necessary in concentrations of about 0.01 per cent. No known toxicity. Polysorbates may increase the absorption of liquid paraffin and other fat-soluble substances and have sometimes been used clinically to treat those with deficient fat absorption.

A.D.I.   0–25mg/kg body weight (1979).

*Typical
Products*   Cakes and cake mixes
              Bread and doughnuts
              Whipped mixes
              Whipped vegetable oil toppings
              Cake icings and fillings
              Ice cream
              Frozen desserts
              Non-dairy coffee whiteners
              Processed powdered food

E440(a)   **Pectin**

Source   Protopectin is a polysaccharide present between the cell walls of plants, cementing them together. During the ripening process of acid fruits (especially apples, plums, bitter oranges and lemons) protopectin accumulates and, as the fruit matures, enzymes break down the protopectin to the softer pectin. Apple residues from cider-making and orange pith are the commercial sources of pectin. Pectin consists mainly of the partial methyl esters of polygalacturonic acid.

Function   Efficient emulsifying and gelling agent in acid media; thickening agent; bodying agent for artificially sweetened beverages; to make syrups for frozen products; stabilizer.

Effects	No real toxicological risks. Large amounts may cause temporary flatulence or intestinal distension, but also reduce blood cholesterol levels.
A.D.I.	Not specified.

Typical Products	Jams
	Jellies
	Marmalades
	Flans
	Puddings
	Desserts
	Water ices
	Ice cream
	Frozen products
	Beverages
	Flavoured yogurts
	Turkish Delight

E440(b)   Amidated pectin

Source	Treatment of pectin (E440a) with ammonia, under alkaline conditions, so that a proportion of the methyl esters are converted to primary amides.
Function	Emulsifier; stabilizer; gelling agent especially for low-sugar gels; thickener.
Effects	No adverse effects are known.
A.D.I.	Not specified.

Typical Products	Jams
	Preserves

442 Ammonium phosphatides (Emulsifier YN)

Source   Prepared synthetically.

Function   Stabilizer; emulsifier.

Effects   None known.

A.D.I.   No available information.

Typical Products   Cocoa and chocolate products

Under consideration by the EEC for an 'E' prefix.

E450(a) *di*Sodium dihydrogen diphosphate (*di*Sodium pyrophosphate; DSPP; *di*Sodium dihydrogen pyrophosphate; Acid sodium pryophosphate)

Source   A sodium salt of pyrophosphoric acid. It is prepared by the heat condensation of sodium orthophosphate (in turn made from phosphoric acid).

Function   Buffer; sequestrant; emulsifier; raising agent (for use in conjunction with sodium bicarbonate in flour goods); colour improver; chelating agent (see glossary).
    This additive is not widely used in the United Kingdom.

Effects   Phosphorus, as phosphate, is an essential nutrient present in bones, teeth, blood and cells, and is necessary for fat and protein assimilation and B vitamin digestion. The body can use it most efficiently if it is present in a constant 1:1 ratio with calcium, so it is important that the calcium/phosphate balance is maintained.

In view of the concern expressed that high intakes of phosphates and polyphosphates may be upsetting this balance, in 1982 JECFA recommended that further studies should be carried out on the implications of high dietary intakes of phosphorus.

The main toxicological finding in feeding studies with high levels of phosphates is kidney stones, to which rats are highly susceptible.

A.D.I. 0–70mg/kg body weight (sum of phosphates and polyphosphates).

Typical Processed cheeses
Products Processed meats (e.g. sausages, burgers)
Baking powder
Self-raising flour
Cakes and cake mixes
Frozen potato chips
Instant mashed potatoes

E450(a) *tri*Sodium diphosphate

Source A sodium salt of pyrophosphoric acid.

Function Buffer; sequestrant; emulsifier; colour improver; chelating agent (see glossary).

Effects Phosphorus, as phosphate, is an essential nutrient present in bones, teeth, blood and cells, and is necessary for fat and protein assimilation and B vitamin digestion. The body can use it most efficiently if it is present in a constant 1:1 ratio with calcium, so it is important that the calcium/phosphorus balance is maintained.

227

In view of the concern expressed that high intakes of phosphates and polyphosphates may be upsetting this balance, JECFA in 1982 recommended that further studies should be carried out on the implications of high dietary intakes of phosphorus.

The main toxicological finding in feeding studies with high levels of phosphates is kidney stones, to which rats are highly susceptible.

A.D.I.   Maximum Total Daily Intake (since phosphorus [as phosphate] is an essential nutrient this is more appropriate than an A.D.I.): 0–70mg/kg (sum of phosphates and polyphosphates).

Typical Products   Processed cheeses
Processed meats (e.g. burgers and sausages)

E450(a)   **tetraSodium diphosphate (tetraSodium pyrophosphate)**

Source   A sodium salt of pyrophosphoric acid.

Function   Buffer; emulsifying salt; sequestrant; gelling agent; stabilizer. A special milk-gelling grade of this additive is often used to achieve the desired set body of a dessert whip. It is used to aid rehydration and stabilize colour in dehydrated foods.

Effects   Phosphorus, as phosphate, is an essential nutrient present in bones, teeth, blood and cells, and is necessary for fat and protein assimilation and B vitamin digestion. The body can use it most efficiently if it is present in a constant 1:1 ratio with calcium, so it is important that the calcium/phosphorus balance is maintained.

In view of the concern expressed that high intakes of phosphates and polyphosphates may be upsetting this balance, JECFA in 1982 recommended that further studies should be carried out on the implications of high dietary intakes of phosphorus.

The main toxicological finding in feeding studies with high levels of phosphates is kidney stones, to which rats are highly susceptible.

A.D.I.   Maximum Total Daily Intake (since phosphorus [as phosphate] is an essential nutrient this is more appropriate than an A.D.I.): 0–70mg/kg (sum of phosphates and polyphosphates).

Typical   Cheese spread
Products Processed cheese
Catering whipping cream
Condensed milk
Dried milk products
Pork pies
Frozen turkey meat loaf
Instant dessert whips
Cheesecake mixes
Instant mashed potatoes
Apple pies
Beefburgers, sausages
Tinned ham
Fish fingers
Meat spread

E450(a)   *tetra*Potassium diphosphate

Source   A potassium salt of pyrophosphoric acid.

Function   Emulsifying salt; buffer; sequestrant; stabilizer. Not widely used in the UK.

Effects   Phosphorus, as phosphate, is an essential nutrient present in bones, teeth, blood and cells, and is necessary for fat and protein assimilation and B vitamin digestion. The body can use it most efficiently if it is present in a constant 1:1 ratio with calcium, so it is important that the calcium/phosphorus balance is maintained.

In view of the concern expressed that high intakes of phosphates and polyphosphates may be upsetting this balance, JECFA in 1982 recommended that further studies should be carried out on the implications of high dietary intakes of phosphorus.

The main toxicological finding in feeding studies with high levels of phosphates is kidney stones, to which rats are highly susceptible.

A.D.I.   Maximum Total Daily Intake (since phosphorus [as phosphate] is an essential nutrient this is more appropriate than an A.D.I.): 0–70mg/kg (sum of phosphates and polyphosphates).

Typical Products   Processed meats

E450(b)   *penta*Sodium triphosphate (STPP; Sodium tripolyphosphate)

Source   A sodium salt of triphosphoric acid. Prepared by the heat condensation of sodium orthophosphates.

Function   Emulsifying salt; texturizer; buffer; sequestrant; stabilizer. By using polyphosphates, manufacturers can incorporate water into meat products by enhancing the water-binding ability of muscle proteins (which explains why bacon often seems to disappear in the pan). The declaration of water content will be controlled, see page 24. Polyphosphates are also used for protein substitution (in conjunction with salt) in, for example, comminuted (finely chopped) meats.

Effects   Phosphorus (as phosphate) is an essential nutrient, present in bones, teeth, blood and cells, and is necessary for fat and protein assimilation and B vitamin digestion. The body can use it most efficiently if it is present in an equal ratio with calcium, so it is important that the calcium/phosphorus balance is maintained. Too much phosphate could upset the balance and cause a deficiency of both minerals. When rats are given high levels of phosphates they develop kidney stones (nephrocalcinosis), but man is not considered to have anything approaching the rat's susceptibility.

A.D.I.   Maximum Total Daily Intake (since phosphorus [as phosphate] is an essential nutrient this is more appropriate than an A.D.I.): 0–70mg/kg (sum of phosphates and polyphosphates).

Typical   Processed cheeses
Products   Unsweetened condensed milk
Processed meats (e.g. burgers, re-formed steaks)
Tinned ham and luncheon meat
Beef spread
Pork pies
Processed fish products
Custard powder
Packet cup soup

E450(b)   *penta*Potassium triphosphate (Potassium tripolyphosphate)

Source A potassium salt of triphosphoric acid. Prepared by the heat condensation of potassium ortho-phosphates.

Function Emulsifying salt; texturizer; buffer; sequestrant; stabilizer. This additive is not widely used in the United Kingdom.

Effects Phosphorus (as phosphate) is an essential nutrient present in bones, teeth, blood and cells, and is necessary for fat and protein assimilation and B vitamin digestion. The body can use it most efficiently if it is present in an equal ratio with calcium, so it is important that the calcium/phosphorus balance is maintained. Too much phosphate could upset the balance and cause a deficiency of both minerals. When rats are given high levels of phosphates they develop kidney stones (nephrocalcinosis), but man is not considered to have anything approaching the rat's susceptibility.

A.D.I. Maximum Total Daily Intake (since phosphorus [as phosphate] is an essential nutrient this is more appropriate than an A.D.I.): 0–70mg/kg (sum of phosphates and polyphosphates).

Typical Products Tinned hot dog sausages
Processed meats

E450(c)   Sodium polyphosphates

Source Sodium salts of polyphosphoric acids.

Function   Emulsifying salts; sequestrants; stabilizers; texturizers.

Effects   Phosphorus, as phosphate, is an essential nutrient present in bones, teeth, blood and cells, and is necessary for fat and protein assimilation and B vitamin digestion. The body can use it most efficiently if it is present in a constant 1:1 ratio with calcium, so it is important that the calcium/phosphorus balance is maintained.

In view of the concern expressed that high intakes of phosphates and polyphosphates may be upsetting this balance, the JECFA in 1982 recommended that further studies should be carried out on the implications of high dietary intakes of phosphorus.

The main toxicological finding in feeding studies with high levels of phosphates is kidney stones, to which rats are highly susceptible.

A.D.I.   Maximum Total Daily Intake (since phosphorus [as phosphate] is an essential nutrient this is more appropriate than an A.D.I.): 0–70mg/kg (sum of phosphates and polyphosphates).

Typical   Processed meats (ham, bacon, sausages, burgers,
Products   poultry products)
Processed seafoods (frozen fish fingers/portions,
        breaded scampi)
Tinned custard
Reduced-sugar jam products
Processed cheeses
Frozen turkey meat loaf
Frozen fish fingers and fishcakes
Pork pies

E450(c)   Potassium polyphosphates

Source   Potassium salts of polyphosphoric acids prepared
by the heat condensation of potassium ortho-
phosphates.

Function   Emulsifying salts; stabilizers; sequestrants. This
substance is not widely used in the United
Kingdom.

Effects   Phosphorus, as phosphate, is an essential nutrient
present in bones, teeth, blood and cells, and is
necessary for fat and protein assimilation and B
vitamin digestion. The body can use it most
efficiently if it is present in a constant 1:1 ratio
with calcium, so it is important that the calcium/
phosphorus balance is maintained.

In view of the concern expressed that high
intakes of phosphates and polyphosphates may
be upsetting this balance, JECFA in 1982 recommended that further studies should be carried out
on the implications of high dietary intakes of
phosphorus.

The main toxicological finding in feeding
studies with high levels of phosphates is kidney
stones, to which rats are highly susceptible.

A.D.I.   Maximum Total Daily Intake (since phosphorus
[as phosphate] is an essential nutrient this is more
appropriate than an A.D.I.): 0–70mg/kg (sum of
phosphates and polyphosphates).

Typical   Processed meat products (e.g. burgers and
Products   sausages)
Cheese
Unsweetened condensed milk products

E460   **Microcrystalline cellulose**

Source   The cellulose walls of plant fibres which are chemically fragmented into microscopic crystals.

Function   Non-nutritive bulking agent; binder; anti-caking agent; dietary fibre; hydration aid; emulsion stabilizer; heat stabilizer; alternative ingredient; binder and disintegrant for tablets; carrier and microdispersant for quick drying; cellulose component and for texture modification.

Effects   No adverse effects are known.

A.D.I.   Not specified.

Typical Products
High-fibre bread
Low-calorie cake, biscuits and sweets
Reduced-calorie bread
Imitation Mozzarella cheese
Grated and shredded cheese
Colours, flavours and food acids
Expanded snacks
Imitation spices
Simulated fruit pieces
Dehydrated foods

E460   **Alpha-cellulose (Powdered cellulose)**

Source   The cellulose component of plant cell walls which are disintegrated mechanically to form a pulp and then dried.

Function   Bulking aid; anti-caking agent; binder; dispersant; thickening agent and filter aid; used to assist isinglass finings in clearing of beer, associating with the protein and causing it to flocculate or collect into larger particles and settle.

Effects	None known.
A.D.I.	Not specified.

Typical Products	Beer
	Not permitted in food intended specifically for babies or young children.

E461   **Methylcellulose (Methocel; Cologel)**

Source   Prepared from cellulose by treatment with alkali and methyl chloride.

Function   Emulsifier; stabilizer; thickener; bulking and binding agent; film former and a substitute for water soluble gums. Also used in foods for diabetics, coeliacs or people who are allergic to gluten, or on low calorie diets, or kosher diets. Can function as a fat barrier.

Effects   Methylcellulose reacts and forms complexes in solution with methylhydroxybenzoate (E218) and propylhydroxybenzoate (E217). Excessive amounts could cause flatulence, distension or intestinal obstruction. People with intestinal obstruction should avoid foods containing methylcellulose. It is not know how the presence of the substance in the gut affects the absorption of nutrients.

A.D.I.   No available information.

Typical Products	Frozen bubble and squeak
	Potato waffles
	Beverages
	Special diet food

Bakery fillings
Whipped toppings
Soft drinks
Sauces
Dressings

E463   Hydroxypropylcellulose

Source   Synthetically prepared from cellulose by treatment with alkali and propylene oxide.

Function   Stabilizer in foams and lotions; emulsifier; thickener; suspending agent.

Effects   No adverse effects are known.

A.D.I.   No available information.

Typical Products   Whipped toppings
Glaze on confectionery

E464   Hydroxypropylmethylcellulose (Hypromellose)

Source   Prepared from cellulose by treatment with alkali and methyl chloride and propylene oxide.

Function   Gelling or suspending agent; emulsifier; stabilizer and thickening agent; can function as a fat barrier.

Effects   No adverse effects are known.

A.D.I.   Not stated.

Typical Products	Frozen potato waffles

E465   **Ethylmethylcellulose (Methylethylcellulose)**

Source   Prepared from cellulose.

Function   Emulsifier; foam stabilizer; thickener; suspending agent.

Effects   No adverse effects are known.

A.D.I.   0–25mg/kg body weight.

Typical Products   —

E466   **Carboxymethylcellulose, sodium salt (Carmellose sodium; CMC)**

Source   Prepared by treating cellulose with alkali and monochloroacetic acid.

Function   Thickening agent; texture modification; stabilizer; moisture migration control; gelling agent; non-nutritive bulking agent; prevention of crystal growth, prevention of syneresis (the drawing together of particles in a gel); decreasing fat absorption; foam stabilizer.

Effects   When five healthy male volunteers were given 15g sodium carboxymethylcellulose (7.5 times the A.D.I.) for twenty-three days they experienced no adverse effects. It had no effect on the biochemistry of the blood plasma, red and white blood cells or haemoglobin, urine composition, glucose tolerance, blood cholesterol, etc. The intestine transit time decreased for four of the five and increased for the fifth. Faecal fat increased in four of the men. CMC passes through the food canal without being digested or absorbed into the bloodstream.

A.D.I.   0–25mg/kg body weight.

Typical Products

Packet cheesecake and cake mixes
Icings
Bakery fillings
Fruit bar filling
Lemon pie filling
Meringues
Dips and spreads
Tinned potato salad
Tinned cream soups
Frozen whipped toppings
Whipped topping basis
Sterilized whipping cream
Ice cream
Milk shake
Frozen mousses
Tomato sauces
Salad dressings
Frozen chips
Frozen fish sticks
Batter coating
Low-calorie orange squash
Processed cheese
Cottage cheese
Instant drinks
Custard and dessert puddings
Instant mashed potatoes

E470   **Sodium, potassium and calcium salts of fatty acids (soaps)**

Source   Prepared from fatty acids.

Function   Emulsifiers; stabilizers; anti-caking agents.

Effects   No adverse effects are known.

A.D.I.   Not available.

Typical Products   Packet Black Forest gateau mix
Crispy snacks
Shaped crisps

E471   **Mono- and di-glycerides of fatty acids (Glyceryl monostearate, distearate)**

Source   A normal product of digestion, but prepared for commercial use from glycerin and fatty acids.

Function   Used in cakes to retain the foaming power of egg protein in the presence of fat; emulsifier; stabilizer; thickening agent.

Effects   No adverse effects are known.

A.D.I.   Not limited.

Typical Products   Packet Black Forest gateau mixes
Low-cholesterol margarine
Quick custard mix
Hot chocolate mix
Dried potato cakes
Dehydrated mashed potato
Packet dessert topping

Prepacked cakes
Jam sponge pudding (prepacked)
Shaped crisps
Aerosol cream
Packet savoury meal mix
Mousse mix

E472(a)   **Acetic acid esters of mono- and di-glycerides of fatty acids (Acetylated mono- and di-glycerides; Acetoglycerides; complete and partial glycerol esters)**

Source   Prepared from esters of glycerol and acetic acid.

Function   Emulsifiers, stabilizers; coating agents; texture modifying agents; solvents and lubricants.

Effects   No adverse effects are known.

A.D.I.   Not limited.

Typical Products   Packet cheesecake mix
Packet dessert topping
Packet mousse mix

E472(b)   **Lactic acid esters of mono- and di-glycerides of fatty acids (Lactylated mono- and di-glycerides; Lactoglycerides)**

Source   Prepared from esters of glycerol and lactic acid.

Function   Emulsifiers; stabilizers.

Effects   No adverse effects are known.

A.D.I.	Not limited.

Typical Products	Packet cheesecake mixes Packet dessert topping Packet mousse mix

E472(c)   Citric acid esters of mono- and di-glycerides of fatty acids (Citroglycerides)

Source	Prepared from esters of glycerol and citric acid.
Function	Emulsifiers and stabilizers.
Effects	No adverse effects are known.
A.D.I.	Not limited.

Typical Products	Packet dessert topping

E472(d)   Tartaric acid esters of mono- and di-glycerides of fatty acids

Source	Prepared from esters of glycerol and tartaric acid.
Function	Emulsifiers and stabilizers.
Effects	No adverse effects are known.
A.D.I.	Not limited.

Typical Products	—

E472(e) Mono- and di-acetyltartaric acid esters of mono- and di-glycerides of fatty acids

Source   Prepared from esters of glycerol and tartaric acid.

Function   Emulsifiers; stabilizers.

Effects   No adverse effects are known.

A.D.I.   Not limited.

*Typical
Products*   Hot chocolate mix
                Brown bread rolls
                Frozen pizza
                Gravy granules

E473 Sucrose esters of fatty acids

Source   Prepared from esters of glycerol and sucrose.

Function   Emulsifiers; stabilizers.

Effects   No adverse effects are known.

A.D.I.   No available information.

*Typical
Products*   —

E474 Sucroglycerides

Source   Prepared by the action of sucrose on natural
                triglycerides (from lard, tallow, palm oil, etc.).

243

Function	Emulsifiers; stabilizers.
Effects	Sucroglycerides are hydrolyzed in the food canal to normal dietary constituents prior to absorption. Long- and short-term studies revealed no adverse effects, neither did a study in dogs fed sucrose esters from beef tallow fatty acids.
A.D.I.	0–10mg/kg body weight.
Typical Products	—

E475   Polyglycerol esters of fatty acids

Source	Prepared in the laboratory.
Function	Emulsifiers; stabilizers.
Effects	No adverse effects are known.
A.D.I.	0–25mg/kg body weight.
Typical Products	Packet cheesecake and cake mixes Prepacked sponge pudding Prepacked cakes

476   Polyglycerol esters of polycondensed fatty acids of castor oil (Polyglycerol polyricinoleate)

Source	Prepared from castor oil and glycerol esters.
Function	Emulsifiers; stabilizers; when used with lecithin improve the fluidity of chocolate for coating,

reducing the amount of expensive cocoa butter necessary, allowing a thinner coating of chocolate and maximizing the manufacturers' profit.

Effects	No adverse effects are known.
A.D.I.	0–75mg/kg body weight.

Typical Products	Chocolate-coated biscuits Chocolate-coated cakes Chocolate-coated sweets

Under consideration by the EEC for an 'E' prefix.

E477 Propane-1,2-diol esters of fatty acids (Propylene glycol esters of fatty acids)

Source	Prepared from propylene glycol.
Function	Emulsifiers, stabilizers.
Effects	No adverse effects known.
A.D.I.	0–25mg/kg body weight.

Typical Products	Packet cake mix Instant dessert

478 Lactylated fatty acid esters of glycerol and propane-1,2-diol

Source	Prepared from esters of glycerol and lactic acid.
Function	Emulsifiers; stabilizers; whipping agents; plasticizers; surface-active agents.

Effects	No adverse effects known.
A.D.I.	No available information.

Typical Products	—

Under consideration by the EEC for an 'E' prefix.

E481   Sodium stearoyl-2 lactylate

Source	Prepared from lactic acid.
Function	Stabilizer; emulsifier.
Effects	No adverse effects known.
A.D.I.	0–20mg/kg body weight (temporary).

Typical Products	Biscuits Bread Cakes

E482   Calcium stearoyl-2-lactylate

Source	Prepared from lactic acid.
Function	Emulsifier; stabilizer; whipping aid.
Effects	No adverse effects are known.
A.D.I.	0–20mg/kg body weight.

Typical Products	Gravy granules

E483   Stearyl tartrate

Source   Prepared from tartaric acid.

Function   Stabilizer; emulsifier; flour treatment agent.

Effects   No adverse effects are known.

A.D.I.   0–500ppm.

Typical Products   —

491   Sorbitan monostearate

Source   Prepared synthetically from stearic acid and sorbitol.

Function   Emulsifier; stabilizer; glazing agent.

Effects   No adverse effects are known.

A.D.I.   0–25mg/kg body weight (a group A.D.I. for the sum of the sorbitan esters of lauric, oleic, palmitic and stearic acids).

Typical Products   Packet cake mix
Dried yeast

Under consideration by the EEC for an 'E' prefix.

492   Sorbitan tristearate (Span 65)

Source   Prepared synthetically from stearic acid.

Function   Emulsifier; stabilizer.

Effects	Polysorbates may increase the body's absorption of liquid paraffin and fat-soluble substances.
A.D.I.	0–25mg/kg body weight (a group A.D.I. for the sum of the sorbitan esters of lauric, oleic, palmitic and stearic acids).

Typical Products	Rice 'n' raisin crisp confection
	Under consideration by the EEC for an 'E' prefix.

493   Sorbitan monolaurate (Span 20)

Source	Prepared from sorbitol and lauric acid.
Function	Emulsifier; stabilizer; antifoaming agent.
Effects	No adverse effects are known.
A.D.I.	0–25mg/kg body weight (a group A.D.I. for the sum of the sorbitan esters of lauric, oleic, palmitic and stearic acids).

Typical Products	—
	Under consideration by the EEC for an 'E' prefix.

494   Sorbitan mono-oleate (Span 80)

Source	Prepared synthetically from sorbitol and oleic acid.
Function	Stabilizer; emulsifier.
Effects	No adverse effects are known.

A.D.I.   0–25mg/kg body weight (a group A.D.I. for the sum of the sorbitan esters of lauric, oleic, palmitic and stearic acids).

Typical Products   —

Under consideration by the EEC for an 'E' prefix.

495   Sorbitan monopalmitate (Span 40)

Source   Prepared from sorbitol and palmitic acid.

Function   Oil-soluble emulsifier; stabilizer.

Effects   No adverse effects are known.

A.D.I.   0–25mg/kg body weight (a group A.D.I. for the sum of the sorbitan esters of lauric, oleic, palmitic and stearic acids).

Typical Products   —

Under consideration by the EEC for an 'E' prefix.

500   Sodium carbonate

Source   Although naturally occurring as saline residues deposited from the water of alkaline lakes, sodium carbonate is cheaper to manufacture by the Solvay process or electrolytically from sea or saline lake waters.

Function   Base; used in the malting process of beer-making to remove 'testinic acid' from barley in the steep liquor.

| *Effects* | No adverse effects are known in small doses. Large amounts can corrode the gut and cause gastric upsets and circulation problems. |

A.D.I.   Not limited.

| *Typical Products* | Tinned custard |
| | Beer |

Under consideration by the EEC for an 'E' prefix.

---

500   Sodium hydrogen carbonate (Sodium bicarbonate; Baking soda; Bicarbonate of soda)

Source   Prepared synthetically.

Function   Base; aerating agent; diluent.

Effects   There are no problems with this substance in normal use. Laboratory animals treated with bicarbonate of soda to combat lactic acidosis (the result of the body's inability to clear lactic acid from the blood) died more quickly and frequently than untreated animals. Sodium bicarbonate has been given to patients with cardiac arrest for more than fifty years for lactic acidosis and to treat liver failure, and it has recently been recommended that this practice be halted.

A.D.I.   Not limited.

Typical Products   Tinned custard

Under consideration by the EEC for an 'E' prefix.

---

500   Sodium sesquicarbonate (Trona)

Source   Occurs naturally in saline residues with other minerals formed in the same way, in California, Mexico and Egypt. Prepared also commercially.

Function   Base.

Effects   No adverse effects are known.

A.D.I.   No A.D.I.

Typical Products   —

Under consideration by the EEC for an 'E' prefix.

501   Potassium carbonate and Potassium hydrogen carbonate

Source   Potassium bicarbonate may be prepared by saturating a concentrated solution of potassium carbonate with carbon dioxide.

Function   Base; alkali.

Effects   None known. It is used medicinally for the treatment of gastric hyperacidity. After it has been absorbed, it helps to maintain the alkaline balance of the blood.

A.D.I.   Not limited.

Typical Products   —

Under consideration by the EEC for an 'E' prefix.

503   Ammonium carbonate (Hartshorn)

Source   A mixture of ammonium bicarbonate and ammonium carbonate, obtained by subliming a mixture of ammonium sulphate and calcium carbonate.

Function   Buffer; neutralizing agent; leavening agent.

Effects   Turns into carbon dioxide in the stomach. There may be some alteration of the acid-base balance and pH of the urine.

A.D.I.   Not specified.

Typical Products   Baking powder

Under consideration by the EEC for an 'E' prefix.

503   Ammonium hydrogen carbonate (Ammonium bicarbonate)

Source   Prepared by passing an excess of carbon dioxide through concentrated ammonia water.

Function   Alkali; buffer; aerating agent, raising agent.

Effects   There may be some alteration of the acid-base balance and pH of the urine. It is irritant to mucous membranes and is used medically as an expectorant.

A.D.I.   Not specified.

Typical Products   —

Under consideration by the EEC for an 'E' prefix.

504 Magnesium carbonate (Magnesite)

Source Magnesite occurs naturally in serpentine deposits in Greece and India and replacing dolomite and limestone in Austria, Manchuria, Washington and Quebec. It may be prepared by mixing boiling concentrated solutions of magnesium sulphate and sodium carbonate. The 'heavy' variety is a granular powder; the 'light' variety is a very light fine powder.

Function Alkali; anti-caking agent; acidity regulator; anti-bleaching agent.

Effects Magnesium carbonate is insoluble in water but soluble in dilute acids, and is used pharmaceutically as an antacid and laxative. In the small amounts in which it is used in food it is unlikely to affect the pH balance of the stomach, or produce diarrhoea.

A.D.I. Not limited.

Typical Products Table salt
Icing sugar
Soured cream
Butter
Ice cream
Wafer biscuits

Under consideration by the EEC for an 'E' prefix.

---

507 Hydrochloric acid

Source Produced industrially by the interaction of sodium chloride and sulphuric acid. It is one of the chemicals produced in the stomach to assist the digestive process.

Function   Acid; used in the malting process in beer-making to reduce excess losses of carbohydrate from the germinating barley rootlets, and at the brewery it may be added to the malt slurry to compensate for variations in the water supply to arrive at a beer of consistent quality.

Effects   Although highly corrosive and poisonous in its natural state, used as a processing aid this acid is not present in foods in amounts capable of causing harm.

A.D.I.   Not limited.

Typical Products   Beer

Under consideration by the EEC for an 'E' prefix.

508   **Potassium chloride**

Source   Occurs naturally as a saline residue associated with rock salt, and around volcanic vents.

Function   Gelling agent; salt substitute; dietary supplement; may be added to the malt slurry at the brewery to compensate for variations in the water supply in order to arrive at a beer of consistent quality.

Effects   No problems in food use. It can, in large doses, cause intestinal ulceration, sometimes with haemorrhage perforation. Gastric ulceration may occur with sustained release tablets. Unpleasant taste in solution can cause nausea and vomiting. Potassium salts may have a diuretic effect.

A.D.I.   No A.D.I.

Typical   Salt substitute
Products

Under consideration by the EEC for an 'E' prefix.

---

509   **Calcium chloride**

Source   Obtained as a by-product of the Solvay process and is also a product from natural salt brines.

Function   Sequestrant; firming agent. In brewing may be added to the malt slurry to compensate for variations in the water supply in order to arrive at a beer of consistent quality.

Effects   No adverse effects are known.

A.D.I.   Not limited.

Typical   Tinned red kidney beans
Products   Pickled red cabbage

Under consideration by the EEC for an 'E' prefix.

---

510   **Ammonium chloride**

Source   Prepared synthetically.

Function   Yeast food, especially in the beer stages of the fermentation of the wort in brewing; flavour.

Effects   Ammonium chloride is readily absorbed by the food canal and may decrease the acidity of the urine. It should be avoided by people with imperfect liver or kidney functions.

A.D.I.   Not limited.

Typical Products	—

Under consideration by the EEC for an 'E' prefix.

---

513   Sulphuric acid

Source   Prepared commercially by the 'contact' or 'chamber' process.

Function   Acid; used in the malting process in beer-making to reduce excess losses of carbohydrate from the germinated barley rootlets, and at the brewery sulphuric acid may be added to the malt slurry to compensate for variations in the water supply to arrive at a beer of consistent quality.

Effects   Used as a processing aid, although highly corrosive in its natural state, this acid is present in foods in such minute amounts that it is incapable of causing harm.

A.D.I.   No available information.

Typical Products   Beer

Under consideration by the EEC for an 'E' prefix.

---

514   Sodium sulphate (Glauber's salt)

Source   Occurs naturally as thenardite and mirabilite. The USSR, Canada and the USA are the chief producers.

Function   Diluent; in brewing it may be added to the malt slurry to compensate for variations in the water supply to arrive at a beer of consistent quality.

Effects   Although the healthy body can adapt to a wide range of sodium intake daily, excessive sodium can be dangerous because it is closely linked to the body's water balance. Those at greatest risk are small babies and people suffering with kidney and heart complaints. It is an effective purgative.

A.D.I.   No available information.

Typical Products   —

Under consideration by the EEC for an 'E' prefix.

515   Potassium sulphate

Source   Occurs in nature as a triple sulphate of potassium magnesium and calcium, particularly at Stassfurt in Germany.

Function   Salt substitute for dietetic use.

Effects   No adverse effects are known.

A.D.I.   No available information.

Typical Products   —

Under consideration by the EEC for an 'E' prefix.

516   Calcium sulphate (Gypsum, Plaster of Paris)

Source   A naturally occurring mineral; commercial sources are primarily the USA and France, followed by Spain, Great Britain and Canada.

Function	Firming agent; sequestrant; nutrient; yeast food; inert excipient; may be added to the malt slurry at the brewery to compensate for variations in the water supply in order to arrive at a beer of consistent quality.
Effects	None known.
A.D.I.	Not limited.
Typical Products	Beer

Under consideration by the EEC for an 'E' prefix.

518 Magnesium sulphate (Epsom salts, Epsomite)

Source	Occurs in solution in sea- and mineral-waters and is deposited from the waters of saline lakes and as crusts in limestone caves.
Function	Dietary supplement; firming agent; used in making 'Burton'-style beer, by adjusting the composition of the brewing water to that used by breweries in the Burton-on-Trent area.
Effects	An effective laxative, magnesium is not absorbed to any large extent by the body so that toxicity is not a problem except to people whose kidneys are functioning imperfectly.
A.D.I.	No available information.
Typical Products	—

Under consideration by the EEC for an 'E' prefix.

524   Sodium hydroxide (Caustic soda; Lye)

Source   Manufactured by electrolysis from brine, or precipitated from sodium carbonate and lime solution (Gossage's method).

Function   Base especially to neutralize free fatty acids in the manufacture of food oils, colour solvent; authorized in the manufacture of caramel; oxidizing agent, especially of black olives; used in the malting process of beer-making to remove 'testinic acid' from barley in the steep liquor and, at the brewery, sodium hydroxide may be added to the malt slurry, to compensate for variations in the water supply in order to arrive at a beer of consistent quality.

Effects   Used as a processing aid it is not used in amounts which would be caustic.

A.D.I.   Not limited.

Typical Products   Beer
Jams and preserves
Black olives

Under consideration by the EEC for an 'E' prefix.

525   Potassium hydroxide

Source   Prepared industrially by electolysis of potassium chloride.

Function   Base; oxidizing agent, especially of black olives.

Effects   Used as a processing aid, it is not used in amounts which would be caustic.

A.D.I.   —

Typical Products   Cocoa products
Black olives

Under consideration by the EEC for an 'E' prefix.

526   Calcium hydroxide

Source   Prepared by the hydration of lime.

Function   Firming agent; neutralizing agent; used in the malting process of beer-making to remove 'testinic acid' from barley in the steep liquor and, at the brewery, calcium hydroxide may be added to the malt slurry to compensate for variations in the water supply to arrive at a beer of consistent quality.

Effects   Used as a processing aid it is not used in amounts that would be caustic.

A.D.I.   Not limited.

Typical Products   Beer
Cheese
Cocoa products
Shaped crisps

Under consideration by the EEC for an 'E' prefix.

527   Ammonium hydroxide

Source   Prepared from ammonia gas.

Function   Food colouring diluent and solvent; alkali.

Effects Used as a processing aid, it is highly unlikely to be present in amounts that would be caustic.

A.D.I. Not limited.

Typical Food colours
Products Cocoa products

  Under consideration by the EEC for an 'E' prefix.

528 **Magnesium hydroxide**

Source Occurs in nature as the mineral periclase. It is prepared commercially from magnesite ores.

Function Alkali.

Effects Used as a processing aid, it is not used in amounts that would be caustic.

A.D.I. Not limited.

Typical Cocoa products
Products

  Under consideration by the EEC for an 'E' prefix.

529 **Calcium oxide (Quicklime)**

Source Prepared from limestone.

Function Alkali; nutrient.

Effects Used as a processing aid, it is not used in amounts that would be caustic.

A.D.I. Not limited.

Typical Products	Some cocoa products
	Under consideration by the EEC for an 'E' prefix.

530 Magnesium oxide (Periclase; Native magnesium)

Source A naturally occurring mineral, particularly in rocks which have undergone change brought about by pressure and heat, and it is prepared commercially from magnesite ores. It then has to be specially prepared to be in the right form to absorb water and function as an anti-caking agent.

Function Anti-caking agent; alkali.

Effects None known.

A.D.I. Not limited.

Typical Products Some cocoa products

Under consideration by the EEC for an 'E' prefix.

535 Sodium ferrocyanide (Sodium hexacyanoferrate II)

Source Manufactured synthetically.

Function Anti-caking agent; crystal modifier.

Effects There is a very strong chemical bonding between the iron and cyanide groups which prevents ferrocyanides from being toxic (see 536).

A.D.I.   0–0.025mg/kg body weight.

Typical —
Products

Under consideration by the EEC for an 'E' prefix.

536   **Potassium ferrocyanide (Potassium hexacyanoferrate II)**

Source   Prepared on a commercial scale as a by-product in the purification of coal gas.

Function   Anti-caking agent, especially in table salt. Used to remove excessive metals, especially iron and copper in white and rosé wine production. First a controlled amount of potassium ferrocyanide and then zinc sulphate heptahydrate are added which brings down a blue precipitate of the metals. The process is called 'blue finings'.

Effects   Because the iron and cyanide groups are strongly bonded there is a very low level of toxicity. Nevertheless, ferrocyanides, like nitrates and nitrites (E249–E252), are 'metahaemoglobinants' which means they are capable of converting the haemoglobin in the red blood corpuscles from the ferrous to the ferric states. In the ferric state the haemoglobin is incapable of transporting oxygen.

In streams and lakes, waste ferrocyanide exceeding 2ppm could become irradiated and present a toxicity problem to fish.

A.D.I.   0–0.25mg/kg body weight (calculated as Sodium ferrocyanide).

Typical Products	Some wines

Under consideration by the EEC for an 'E' prefix.

---

540 *di*Calcium diphosphate (*di*Calcium pyrophosphate)

Source Occurs in nature as the mineral monetite, also prepared synthetically.

Function Neutralizing agent; dietary supplement; buffering agent; yeast food. Some countries use it as a mineral supplement in cereals and other foods, but it is not used in this way in the United Kingdom.

Effects Little dicalcium diphosphate is absorbed by the intestines, and there is little danger of any adverse reaction.

A.D.I. Maximum Total Daily Intake (since phosphorus [as phosphate] is an essential nutrient this is more appropriate than an A.D.I.): 0–70mg/kg body weight (sum of phosphates and polyphosphates).

Typical Products Some cheeses, especially processed cheeses
Shaped crisps

Under consideration by the EEC for an 'E' prefix.

---

541 Sodium aluminium phosphate, acidic (SAP)

Source Prepared from high-purity phosphoric acid.

Function Aerator; acidulant (raising agent) in flour confectionery.

Effects   Sodium aluminium phosphate has been considered by the toxicological committees on the basis of its aluminium, rather than its phosphates component. Aluminium poses a problem because of the evidence that there is an accumulation of it in the cells of the nervous system could be potentially toxic, and responsible for Parkinson-type diseases and senile dementia. However, a high aluminium content may have adverse effects on the metabolism of phosphorus, calcium or fluoride and may induce or intensify skeletal abnormalities.

A.D.I.   0–6mg/kg body weight (temporary, allocated to sodium aluminium phosphates).

Typical Products   Cake and cake mixes
Scones
Enrobing batters
Pancake mixes
Processed cheeses

Under consideration by the EEC for an 'E' prefix.

---

541   Sodium aluminium phosphate, basic

Source   Prepared from high-purity phosphoric acid.

Function   Emulsifying salt in processed cheese manufacture in America.

Effects   Sodium aluminium phosphate has been considered by the toxicological committees on the basis of its aluminium rather than its phosphate component. Aluminium poses a problem because of the evidence that an accumulation of it in the cells of the nervous system could be potentially toxic, and responsible for Parkinson-type diseases and senile dementia. However, a high aluminium content may have adverse effects on the metabolism of phosphorus, calcium or fluoride and may induce or intensify skeletal abnormalities.

A.D.I. 0–6mg/kg body weight (temporary, allocated to sodium aluminium phosphates).

Typical Products Individually wrapped sliced processed cheese

Under consideration by the EEC for an 'E' prefix.

542   Edible bone phosphate

Source The degreased steam-extract from animal bones. It is calcium phosphate in an impure state, although the impurities do not affect its activity, being of biological origin.

Function Anti-caking agent; mineral supplement; filler in tablet making. A product peculiar to Britain.

Effects None known.

A.D.I. —

Typical Products —

Under consideration by the EEC for an 'E' prefix.

544   Calcium polyphosphates

Source Calcium salts of polyphosphoric acids. Manufactured by the heat condensation of calcium orthophosphate.

Function   Emulsifying salts — have an action on milk proteins which prevents processed cheeses from separating out; mineral supplements; calcium source in instant milk-based desserts; firming agents. This substance is not used in the United Kingdom.

Effects   Calcium and phosphorus are both essential nutrients present in bones and teeth, and as long as they are used in a constant ratio there should be no problem.

A.D.I.   0–70mg/kg body weight (expressed as phosphorus).

Typical Products   —

Under consideration by the EEC for an 'E' prefix.

545   **Ammonium polyphosphates**

Source   Ammonium salts of polyphosphoric acids.

Function   Emulsifiers; emulsifying salts; sequestrants; yeast foods; stabilizers.

Effects   Phosphorus as phosphate is an essential nutrient present in bones, teeth, blood and cells. It is necessary for fat and protein assimilation and B vitamin absorption. The body can use it most efficiently if it is present in a constant ratio with calcium.

   In view of the concern expressed that high intakes of phosphates and polyphosphates may be upsetting this balance, JECFA, in 1982, recommended that further studies should be carried out on the implications of high dietary intakes of phosphorus.

A.D.I.　　0–70mg/kg body weight (expressed as phosphorus).

Typical Products　　Cheeses

Under consideration by the EEC for an 'E' prefix.

551　　Silicon dioxide (Silicea, Silica, Lucilite)

Source　　Silicon dioxide is the commonest rock-forming mineral and sand is composed mainly of small grains of quartz or flint, both of which are silicon dioxide. For use in foods, quartz is further processed to produce a microcellular powder, a granular gel form and a colloidal form by further hydrolysis.

Function　　Suspending and anti-caking agent; thickener and stabilizer in suspensions and emulsions, including wine. Used to assist isinglass finings in clearing of beer by associating with the protein and causing it to flocculate and settle, and as a filtration aid when suspended yeast is filtered from 'green' beer.

Effects　　No adverse effects are known in food use because it is so inert.

A.D.I.　　Not limited.

Typical Products　　Shaped crisps
Beer
Wine in which total use of all silicates should not exceed 2,000mg/l of beer

Under consideration by the EEC for an 'E' prefix.

552 Calcium silicate

Source
A naturally occurring mineral in impure limestones known as wollastonite. Many different forms of calcium silicate are known with various percentages of water or crystallization. Commercial calcium silicate (*Micro-Cel Sil-Ca* and *Silene*) is prepared from lime and diatomaceous earth under carefully controlled conditions.

To be an effective anti-caking agent, a hydrated silicate has to be precipitated and subsequently dried to ensure an 'active' material that will attract moisture.

Function
Anti-caking agent; in pharmacology as an antacid; glazing, polishing and release agent (sweets); dusting agent (chewing gum); coating agent (rice); suspending agent.

Effects
No adverse effects are known. It is used pharmaceutically as an antacid.

A.D.I.
Not limited.

Typical Products
Salt
Garlic and onion salt
Icing sugar
Sweets
Rice
Chewing gum

Under consideration by the EEC for an 'E' prefix.

553(a)   Magnesium silicate, synthetic and Magnesium trisilicate

Source
Magnesium silicate is a synthetic compound of magnesium oxide and silicon dioxide, or can be prepared from sodium silicate and magnesium sulphate. Magnesium trisilicate occurs in nature as the minerals meerschaum, parasepiolite and sepiolite.

To be an effective anti-caking agent, a hydrated silicate is precipitated and subsequently dried to ensure an 'active' material that will attract moisture.

Function
Anti-caking agent and tablet excipient and as an antacid in pharmacology; glazing, polishing and release agent (sweets); dusting agent (chewing gum); coating agent (rice).

Effects
Magnesium trisilicate is non-toxic even in very large doses. It has absorbent and antacid properties and the action continues slowly for some time.

A.D.I.
Not specified.

Typical Products
Salt
Garlic and onion salt
Icing sugar
Sweets
Rice
Chewing gum

Under consideration by the EEC for an 'E' prefix.

553(b)   Talc (French chalk; Magnesium hydrogen metasilicate)

Source   A naturally occurring mineral, worked in the USA, France, Italy, Canada, etc.

Function   Release agent; anti-caking agent; chewing gum component; filtering aid and dusting powder.

Effects   There have been reports of links between talc and stomach cancer.

A.D.I.   Not specified.

Typical Products   —

Under consideration by the EEC for an 'E' prefix.

554   Aluminium sodium silicate (Sodium aluminosilicate)

Source   Naturally occurring mineral, known as analcite and natrolite and also prepared synthetically by processes starting with quartz and gibbsite.

Function   Anti-caking agent.

Effects   Aluminium salts can be absorbed from the intestines and concentrated in various human tissues, including bone, the parathyroid and the brain. Aluminium has been shown to be neurotoxic (damaging nerves) in rabbits and cats, and high concentrations have been detected in the brain tissue of patients with Alzheimer's disease (senile dementia). Various reports have suggested that high aluminium intakes may be harmful to some patients with bone disease or kidney impairment.

271

A.D.I.	Not limited.

Typical Products	Packet noodles Salt Non-dairy creamers Chewing gum Icing sugar Cocoa powders and milk powders for vending machines

Under consideration by the EEC for an 'E' prefix.

556 Aluminium calcium silicate (Calcium aluminium silicate)

Source Naturally occurring mineral, known as scolecite and heulandite.

Function Anti-caking agent.

Effects Aluminium salts can be absorbed from the intestines and concentrated in various human tissues, including bone, the parathyroid and the brain. Aluminium has been shown to be neurotoxic (damaging nerves) in rabbits and cats, and high concentrations have been detected in the brain tissue of patients with Alzheimer's disease (senile dementia). Various reports have suggested that high aluminium intakes may be harmful to some patients with bone disease or kidney impairment.

A.D.I. No A.D.I. allocated.

Typical Products	Salt Non-dairy creamers Chewing gum

Under consideration by the EEC for an 'E' prefix.

558   Bentonite (Bentonitum; Soap clay)

Source

A particular clay deposit occurring in thin beds in the western USA, believed to result from the decomposition of volcanic ash.

Function

Anti-caking agent; clarifying agent, especially of wine; filtration aid when suspended yeast is filtered from 'green' beer; suspending and emulsifying agent.

Effects

No adverse effects are known.

A.D.I.

Not allocated.

Typical Products

Beer
Wine

Under consideration by the EEC for an 'E' prefix.

559   Kaolin, heavy, and Kaolin, light (Aluminium silicate)

Source

Occurs in nature as an altered mineral in granite, particularly in Cornwall, the USA, France, China and Malaysia.

Function

Anti-caking agent; clarifying agent, especially of wine.

Effects

No adverse effects are known.

A.D.I.

Not limited.

Typical Products	Wine
	Under consideration by the EEC for an 'E' prefix.

570 **Stearic acid**

Source	Naturally occurring fatty acid found in all animal fats and vegetable oils. Prepared synthetically for commercial use.
Function	Anti-caking agent.
Effects	No adverse effects are known.
A.D.I.	Not allocated.

Typical Products	—
	Under consideration by the EEC for an 'E' prefix.

572 **Magnesium stearate**

Source	Prepared synthetically from commercial stearic acid.
Function	Anti-caking agent; emulsifier; release agent.
Effects	No adverse effects are known from the consumption of this additive, but accidental inhalation of the powder can be harmful.
A.D.I.	Not limited.

Typical Products	Sweets made by direct compression
	Under consideration by the EEC for an 'E' prefix.

575   D-Glucono-1,5-lactone (Glucono delta-lactone)

Source   Prepared by oxidation of glucose.

Function   Acid; sequestrant. In the dairy industry prevents milkstone formation (deposits of magnesium and calcium phosphates etc., when milk is heated to a high temperature); in breweries prevents beerstone formation.

Effects   No adverse effects are known.

A.D.I.   0–50mg/kg body weight (calculated as gluconic acid from all sources).

Typical Products   Packet cake mix

Under consideration by the EEC for an 'E' prefix.

576   Sodium gluconate

Source   Prepared synthetically; the sodium salt of gluconic acid.

Function   Sequestrant; dietary supplement.

Effects   No adverse effects are known.

A.D.I.   0–50mg/kg body weight (calculated as gluconic acid from all sources).

Typical Products   —

Under consideration by the EEC for an 'E' prefix.

577   Potassium gluconate

Source   Prepared synthetically; the potassium salt of gluconic acid.

Function   Sequestrant.

Effects   No adverse effects are known.

A.D.I.   0–50mg/kg body weight (calculated as gluconic acid from all sources).

Typical Products   —

Under consideration by the EEC for an 'E' prefix.

578   Calcium gluconate

Source   Prepared synthetically; calcium salt prepared from gluconic acid.

Function   Buffer; firming agent; sequestrant.

Effects   No adverse effects are known.

A.D.I.   0–50mg/kg body weight (calculated as gluconic acid from all sources).

Typical Products   —

Under consideration by the EEC for an 'E' prefix.

620   L-Glutamic acid

Source   A naturally occurring amino acid of great importance in the nitrogen metabolism of plants and animals, but prepared commercially by the fermentation of a carbohydrate solution by a bacterium, e.g. *Micrococcus glutamicus*. Several other methods exist.

Function   Dietary supplement; flavour enhancer; salt substitute.

Effects   In the same way as monosodium glutamate (621) was thought to cause 'Chinese restaurant syndrome', it was supposed that glutamic acid might cause similar problems and it is still considered inadvisable for young children.

The use of glutamate in baby foods in the United States was discontinued voluntarily in 1970 when it was revealed that the amount of glutamate required to induce damage to the immature brain (500mg/kg body weight) was not too different from the 130mg/kg body weight from a 4½ oz jar of baby food.

A.D.I.   0–120mg/kg body weight.

Typical Products   —

Under consideration by the EEC for an 'E' prefix.

621   **monoSodium glutamate (Sodium hydrogen L-glutamate; Aji-no-moto; MSG; Accent; Mejing; Ve-Tsin)**

Source   monoSodium glutamate is the sodium salt of glutamic acid (620). It is an amino acid (several amino acids together make up a protein). The various forms of glutamic acid are referred to as 'glutamates'. Glutamate is a common substance widely found in plant and animal tissues. It occurs especially in foods such as meat, fish, poultry and milk. Human breast milk contains about 22mg of glutamate per 100ml milk, which is ten times as much as in cow's milk.

Early Japanese cooks learnt from experience that foods flavoured with stock made from a seaweed called *Laminaria japonica* tasted delicious. The active substance was isolated in 1908 by a professor at Tokyo University, Kikunae Ikeda, and found to be glutamic acid. He differentiated it from the other four basic tastes of sweet, sour, salty and bitter, and called it '*umami*', roughly translated as 'deliciousness'.

Today 90 per cent is manufactured by fermentation using molasses from cane or beet sugar, and 10 per cent in South-East Asia from sago and tapioca starch, or from plant proteins rich in glutamic acid such as wheat protein and sugar beet.

Function

Interesting sensory work done in Japan shows that the *umami* taste is additional to the four basic tastes. Stocks made from fish or meat come closest to the *umami* taste, while stocks made from vegetables fall much closer within the sweet, sour, bitter or salty areas. When the two are combined there is a 'synergistic effect', the one enormously enhancing the other to a position close to the *umami* one. The interplay of the protein stock with the glutamic acid of the vegetables produces an increase in flavour up to eight times the properties of the ingredients.

MSG is widely used as a flavour enhancer to increase the palatability of proteinaceous foods. It may be a useful ingredient for those needing to reduce their sodium intake, since the larger the amount of monosodium glutamate used, the less salt is required, because sodium is about 13 per cent of MSG by weight but 40 per cent of table salt. Some Chinese takeaway meals contain MSG in quantities of 5–10g.

Effects

The 'Umami Information Centre' is confident that MSG is safe for human intake. It says that research on humans as well as laboratory animals, including mice, rats, hamsters, rabbits, dogs and monkeys, overwhelmingly indicates that MSG taken in reasonable amounts produces no cause for concern. In infant mice, the most susceptible species known, dietary feeding of about 10,000 times the equivalent daily intake level of man produced no harmful effects.

Glutamate does not cross the placenta to reach the developing fetus but once consumed by babies from breast milk it is readily metabolized. The link between monosodium glutamate and the 'Chinese Restaurant Syndrome' first described in 1968 by Dr Robert Ho Man Kwok now seems to be rather tenuous. The symptoms of the syndrome occur after eating meals and consist of a tightening of the jaw muscles, numbness of the neck, chest and hands, thirst and nausea, palpitations, dizziness, fainting, pounding, vice-like headache, and a cold sweat around the face and armpits. Yet, when people who said they suffered from CRS were given drinks with and without MSG they experienced symptoms each time. Orange juice, tomato juice and cold coffee were just as effective as MSG in inducing the reactions, and it is suggested that these people may have sensitive nerve endings in the gullet which transmit the stimulus to the arms and chest. Although uncomfortable, the symptoms are neither long-lasting nor serious.

Despite these safety assurances, experiments on young mice, rats, rabbits, guinea pigs, hamsters and rhesus monkeys showed that MSG caused damage to brain cells. This was true in both infant and adult animals, but adults were only susceptible in much higher doses. Another experiment showed that, whereas exposure to MSG caused mature but not young brain cells to die, the action was dependent on a lack of calcium.

The use of glutamate in baby foods in the United States was voluntarily discontinued in 1970 when it was revealed that the amount of glutamate required to induce damage to the immature brain (500mg/kg body weight) was not too different from the 130mg/kg body weight in a 4½ oz jar of baby food.

It looks as though a consumption of not more than 2g per day will cause no problems in all but the most sensitive people.

A.D.I. 0–120mg/kg body weight.

Typical Products

Packet snacks
Chilli sauce
Frozen potato waffles
Pork pies
Pork sausages
Packet soup and quick soups
Flavoured noodles
Processed cheese preparations
Tinned beans, sweetcorn and mushrooms
Miso ⎫ Japanese fermented juices
Tamari ⎭ rich in natural MSG
Codex permitted use in food:
Cooked cured ham 2g/kg expressed as glutamic acid
Cooked cured pork shoulder 2g/kg expressed as glutamic acid

Cooked cured chopped meat 5g/kg expressed as glutamic acid

Luncheon meat 5g/kg expressed as glutamic acid

Bouillons and consommés 10g/kg singly or in combination with glutamic acid and its salts on a ready-to-eat basis

---

622   Potassium hydrogen L-glutamate (*mono*Potassium glutamate)

Source   Prepared synthetically.

Function   Flavour enhancer; salt substitute.

Effects   Sometimes nausea, vomiting, diarrhoea and abdominal cramps may occur, although there is usually little toxicity of potassium salts when taken by mouth in healthy individuals, as potassium is rapidly excreted in the urine. Potassium could be harmful for those with impaired kidneys. Not to be given to babies under 12 weeks old.

A.D.I.   —

Typical Products   Sodium-free condiments

Under consideration by the EEC for an 'E' prefix.

---

623   Calcium dihydrogen di-L-glutamate

Source   Prepared synthetically.

Function   Flavour enhancer; salt substitute.

Effects   None known, but not to be given to babies under 12 weeks old.

A.D.I.   0–120mg/kg body weight.

---

*Typical
Products*   Dietetic foods
Codex permitted use in food:
Bouillons and consommés 10g/kg singly or in
    combination with glutamic acid (620) and its
    salts

Under consideration by the EEC for an 'E' prefix.

---

627   **Guanosine 5'-(*di*Sodium phosphate)
(Sodium guanylate)**

Source   The sodium salt of 5'guanylic acid, a widely-
occurring nucleotide (isolated from sardines and
yeast extract), prepared synthetically for
commercial use.

Function   Flavour enhancer.

Effects   No adverse effects are known, but prohibited in
or on foods intended for babies or young
children. People suffering from conditions such
as gout, which require the avoidance of purines,
are recommended to avoid this substance.

A.D.I.   Not specified.

---

*Typical
Products*   Precooked fried rice snacks
Crisps
Gravy granules
Codex permitted use in food:
Luncheon meat 500mg/kg expressed as the acid
Cooked cured pork shoulder 500mg/kg expressed
    as the acid
Cooked cured ham 500mg/kg expressed as the
    acid

Cooked cured chopped meat 500mg/kg expressed
  as the acid
Bouillons and consommés

Under consideration by the EEC for an 'E' prefix.

---

631 Inosine 5'-(*di*Sodium phosphate) (Sodium 5'-inosinate)

Source   The disodium salt of inosinic acid (muscle inosinic acid) which can be prepared from meat extract and dried sardines. It was originally isolated from Japanese bonito (a tuna-like fish), small dried flakes of which were often added to improve the flavour of soups.

Function   Flavour enhancer.

Effects   No adverse effects are known, but prohibited in or on foods specially made for babies and young children. People suffering from conditions such as gout which require the avoidance of purines, should avoid this substance.

A.D.I.   Not specified.

Typical Products
Precooked dried rice snacks
Some crisps
Gravy granules
Codex permitted use in food:
Luncheon meat 500mg/kg expressed as the acid
Cooked cured pork shoulder 500mg/kg expressed
  as the acid
Cooked cured ham 500mg/kg expressed as the
  acid
Cooked cured chopped meat 500mg/kg expressed
  as the acid
Bouillons and consommés

Under consideration by the EEC for an 'E' prefix.

635 Sodium 5'-ribonucleotide

Source   A mixture of *di*Sodium guanylate (627) and disodium inosinate (631).

Function   Flavour enhancer.

Effects   No adverse effects are known, but not permitted in foods specially prepared for babies or young children. People suffering from conditions such as gout, which require the avoidance of purines, should avoid this substance.

A.D.I.   Not specified.

Typical Products
Frozen croquette potatoes
Potato waffles
Mini-waffles

Under consideration by the EEC for an 'E' prefix.

636 Maltol

Source   A naturally occurring substance found in the bark of young larch trees, pine needles, chicory wood, tars, oils and roasted malt. Also obtained chemically by alkaline hydrolysis of streptomycin salt.

Function   Flavouring agent, to impart a 'freshly baked' smell and flavour to bread and cakes. Synthetic flavouring agent for coffee, fruit, maple, nut and vanilla flavours.

Effects   None known.

A.D.I.   0–1mg/kg body weight.

Typical   Bread
Products Cakes
     Ice cream
     Chewing gum
     Drinks
     Jams

     Under consideration by the EEC for an 'E' prefix.

---

637   Ethyl maltol

Source   Chemically prepared from maltol.

Function Flavouring to impart a sweet taste and flavour-enhancer.

Effects   No adverse effects are known.

A.D.I.   0–2mg/kg body weight.

Typical   —
Products

     Under consideration by the EEC for an 'E' prefix.

---

900   Dimethylpolysiloxane (Simethicone; Dimethicone)

Source   A chemically manufactured mixture of liquid dimethylpolysiloxane and silicon gel or silicon dioxide.

Function Water repellent; anti-foaming agent in curing

solutions, wine fermentation, skimmed milk, sugar distillation; chewing gum base; anti-caking agent. In the brewing industry in Britain a strain of yeast is added to the fermented wort to ferment the top and form a 'head'. Dimethylpolysiloxane in dilute solution is added at the start of fermentation to inhibit excessive yeast-head formation. This also increases the working capacity of the fermentation vessels.

Effects   As long as the additive does not contain formaldehyde, a (possible) carcinogen, it is safe. Dimethylpolysiloxane used as a food additive may legally contain up to 1,000mg/kg formaldehyde.

A.D.I.   0–1.5mg/kg body weight (this A.D.I. applies only to compounds with a relative molecular mass in the range of 200–300).

Typical Products

Jams
Pineapple juice
Molasses
Soft drinks
Syrups
Soups
Chewing gum
Frozen vegetables

Products containing dimethylpolysiloxane may also contain formaldehyde in additives use up to 1,000mg/kg.
Under consideration by the EEC for an 'E' prefix.

---

901   **Beeswax, white, and Beeswax, yellow**

Source   A naturally occurring product from the bee

honeycomb. White beeswax is the bleached and purified form.

Function Glazing and polishing agent; release agent; also used in fruit and honey flavourings for beverages, ice cream, baked goods and honey.

Effects Beeswax was formerly used to treat diarrhoea and has been used as a repository for slow-release tablets. Resins in the wax occasionally cause hypersensitivity reactions.

A.D.I. No available information.

Typical Products Diluents for food colours and glazes
Baked goods/confectionery

Under consideration by the EEC for an 'E' prefix.

---

903 Carnauba wax

Source A yellow to light-brown wax obtained from the surface of leaves of *Copernicia cerifera*, the Brazilian wax palm. The crude wax is yellow or dirty green, brittle and very hard.

Function Glazing and polishing agent for sugar confectionery. It enhances the hardness of other waxes and increases their lustre. Used in cosmetic materials like depilatories and deodorant sticks.

Effects Skin sensitivity or irritation is infrequent.

A.D.I. No available information.

Typical Products *Only permitted in chocolate products such as in*:
Sugar confectionery

Chocolate confectionery

Under consideration by the EEC for an 'E' prefix.

904   Shellac

Source

Shellac is a substance obtained from the resin produced by the lac insect (*Laccifer lacca*, a member of the *Lacciferidae*) related to mealy bugs and scale insects belonging to the *Coccoidea*. It is a native of India. Four commercial grades are produced by different chemical processes. One method mixes shellac resin with small amounts of arsenic trisulphide (for colour) and rosin. White shellac is free of arsenic.

Function

Glazing agent and polish up to 0.4 per cent.

Effects

No significant reports of adverse effects, although it may cause skin irritation.

A.D.I.

No available information.

Typical Products

Cake decorations
Sweets
Fizzy orange drink
Sugar strands

Under consideration by the EEC for an 'E' prefix.

905   Mineral hydrocarbons

Source

Distillates of petroleum.

Function

Polishes, glazing agents, sealing agents; in confectionery, ingredient for chewing gum;

defoaming agent in processing of sugar beet and yeast; coating for fresh fruit and vegetables; lubricant and binder for capsules and tablets supplying small amounts of flavour, spice, condiments and vitamins. Lubricant in food-processing equipment and meat-packing plants. Allowed up to 2,000ppm as a release agent.

Effects   May inhibit absorption of digestive fats and fat-soluble vitamins, and has a mild laxative effect. There has been some suspicion that liquid paraffin may be partly responsible for bowel cancer. Excessive dosage may result in anal seepage and irritation.

A.D.I.   Not specified.

Typical Products   Dried fruit (to prevent sugaring of berries and clouding of film bags)
Citrus fruit
Sugar confectionery
Chewing gum
Processed cheese rind
Eggs (through dipping or spraying for preserving, which must be declared)

Under consideration by the EEC for an 'E' prefix.

907   Refined microcrystalline wax

Source   Prepared by solution of the heavy fraction of petroleum by dewaxing or de-oiling methods.

Function   Chewing gum ingredient; polishing and release agent; stiffening agent and used for tablet coating.

Effects   The unrefined form is a possible human

carcinogen and the refined form used as a food additive may also be carcinogenic.

A.D.I.	No available information.

Typical Products	—

Under consideration by the EEC for an 'E' prefix.

920 L-cysteine hydrochloride and L-cysteine hydrochloride monohydrate

Source	A diamer of L-cysteine, a naturally occurring amino acid, and manufactured from animal hair and chicken feathers. In China it is made from human hair.
Function	Improving agent for flour, other than wholemeal. Flavour, especially chicken flavour. Also used in shampoo.
Effects	None known.
A.D.I.	No available information.

Typical Products	Flour and bakery products Chicken stock cubes

Under consideration by the EEC for an 'E' prefix.

924 Potassium bromate

Source	Prepared synthetically.
Function	Flour-maturing or -improving agent. It has an

effect on the proteins which make up the gluten in the wheat flour. When the wheat flour is mixed with water the potassium bromate is activated and helps the proteins retain the carbon dioxide gas generated by the yeast during fermentation. The result is a softer, lighter loaf with a good eating quality.

Used in the malting process in beer-making to reduce excess losses of carbohydrate from the germinated barley rootlets. An additional function of the potassium bromate is to control protein degradation within the malting barley and thus reduce the levels of nitrogen in the wort.

Effects In strong concentrations can cause nausea, vomiting, severe abdominal pain, diarrhoea and even convulsions, but, used as a processing aid, even the detectable residue left in beer would not have serious consequences.

A.D.I. 0–75mg/kg body weight (temporary).

Typical Products Bread

Under consideration by the EEC for an 'E' prefix.

925   Chlorine

Source Found in the earth's crust and in seawater, it is a greenish-yellow gas with a suffocating odour. Produced on a large scale by electrolysis.

Function Antibacterial and antifungal preservative; bleaching, ageing and oxidizing agent.

Effects A powerful irritant, which is dangerous to inhale. Bleaching of flour has never been demonstrated to be 100 per cent safe. The process takes its toll of flour nutrients and destroys much of the vitamin E content. The chlorine used in drinking water often contains carcinogenic carbon tetrachloride, a contaminant formed during the production process. Chlorination has also been found to sometimes form undesirable carbon 'ring' compounds in water, such as toluene, xylene and styrene, the suspected carcinogen observed in drinking-water treatment works in the Mid-West of the USA.

A.D.I.	No A.D.I.

Typical Products	Flour
	Under consideration by the EEC for an 'E' prefix.

926   Chlorine dioxide (Chlorine peroxide)

Source	Prepared synthetically by one of a number of methods: from chlorine and sodium chlorite; from potassium chlorate and sulphuric acid; or by passing nitrogen dioxide through a column of sodium chlorate.
Function	Bleaching and improving and oxidizing agent for flour; bleaching agent for fats and oils, beeswax, etc.; purification of water; taste and odour control of water; oxidizing agent; bactericide and antiseptic.
Effects	The gas is highly irritating to the mucous membranes of the respiratory tract but, because it is a processing aid, there are only harmless tiny residues remaining in the flour. Bleaching of flour

has never been demonstrated to be 100 per cent safe. It takes its toll of flour nutrients and destroys much of the vitamin E. Chlorine dioxide was admitted in place of nitrogen trichloride which was found to produce fits in dogs and was therefore considered of doubtful safety for man. Chlorine reacts violently with organic materials.

A.D.I.   0–30mg/kg body weight (conditional).

Typical Products   Flour

Under consideration by the EEC for an 'E' prefix.

927   Azodicarbonamide (Azoformamide; Azo dicarboxilic acid; Azo bisformamide)

Source   Prepared synthetically.

Function   Flour-improving or -maturing agent to improve the tolerance of bread dough under a wide range of fermentation conditions.

Effects   No adverse effects are known.

A.D.I.   Not stated.

Typical Products   Flour

There is no evidence of its use in the UK.

Under consideration by the EEC for an 'E' prefix.

Appendix I
An Introduction to the Safety Assessment (Toxicity) of Additives
by R. D. Combes, PhD (London), MIBiol

The term 'toxic' is derived from the Greek word 'toxon' which means 'arrow poison'. This etymological connection is due to the fact that toxicology developed first along the lines of legal or forensic medicine. The legal connection has more recently shifted towards regulatory decision-making processes concerned with legislation for the use of chemicals in society. Nowadays we tend to think of toxicology as the study of the adverse effects of outside influences — be they radiations or chemicals — on the normal body functions.

The change in emphasis has been prompted primarily by the rapid growth of the chemical industry. Several thousands of chemical substances are in regular use throughout the world, many with unknown toxicological effects. With this development has come an awareness that, in addition to effects occurring rapidly (short-term, acute or sub-acute effects) such as poisoning, chemicals can exert changes which arise some considerable time after exposure (chronic effects). The latter can occur later on in the same generation (e.g. cancer) or in later generations (birth defects and inherited diseases), the consequences of which may not become apparent for several hundreds of years. This is because they are due to alterations that may not be reflected immediately in that chemical (the genetic material, DNA) which is present in the chromosomes in all the body cells and which determines all our characteristics. Chronic effects are often due to continuous exposure to small amounts of chemical over long periods of time, a situation which occurs when we eat food and from any constituents which it contains. Unfortunately most people seem to be more concerned about the immediate consequences of chemicals where the link between exposure and side-effects is more obvious.

Toxicological assessment of chemicals involves three main procedures, all of which are designed to minimize possible adverse effects on the human population:

(1) toxicity testing
(2) data evaluation and risk benefit analysis
(3) legislation regulating manufacture, handling and usage to either ban or limit levels of exposure or to lay down specifications for contents of samples.

In the case of food additives this is carried out by the Food Advisory Committee (FAC) which reports to the government. Food additive legislation has advanced considerably with the publication of the 1987 report on colourings by the FAC (*Final Report on the Review of the Colouring Matter in Food Regulations*, FdAC/REP/4, Ministry of Agriculture Fisheries and Food, published by Her Majesty's Stationery Office). Although the committee recognizes that colourings still have an important function in improving the appearance of foods, its latest set of recommendations are designed to lead to a significant decrease in the amounts of colourings consumed in the diet.

If these suggestions become law, such a reduction in the levels of food dyes will be achieved mainly by: (a) the introduction of statutory limits on amounts of colours added to foods; (b) the banning of colours for which there is insufficient evidence of safety; (c) resisting the future addition of colourings to foods that currently lack them; and (d) the adoption of tighter controls on the incorporation of dyes into foods and on their use for external marking of foods. Also, it is recommended that steps should be taken to obtain up-to-date estimates of the levels of consumption of colours so that the potential hazards of ingesting them can be assessed more meaningfully.

As far as human hazard is concerned, toxicity testing can be undertaken during or after exposure (retrospectively) by looking at groups of people which have been exposed to particular chemicals. This is called epidemiology, and it attempts to see whether such exposed groups exhibit any adverse effect any more frequently than groups not exposed to the chemical.

However, although epidemiology involves detection of direct toxicity to humans, it cannot be used to predict toxic hazard before exposure takes place. Moreover, it is difficult to ascribe effects specifically to a particular chemical due to the complications of using different individuals. For these reasons it is unlikely that a harmful food additive will be identified by this means. However, epidemiology has proved useful in the identification of certain toxic hazards, providing guidance on the possible ways in which exposure of humans takes place. Thus epidemiology cannot be used to test new chemicals; this can only be done by intentionally exposing test organisms and observing the effects resulting.

Although such test organisms can include man, ethical considerations have predominantly resulted in the use of animals for this purpose. More recently other organisms are being used as alternatives to animals. In fact there has been, and is currently, an enormous amount of research into developing useful testing procedures which reduce or eliminate the use of man and other higher animals. This work has led to four main general conclusions:

(1) Every substance can be toxic under certain conditions of exposure.
(2) There is no way of predicting with any certainty from the results of testing whether or not a chemical will be toxic to man — ABSOLUTE SAFETY CAN NEVER BE GUARANTEED.
(3) Toxicity is not a property unique to substances created and produced by man. Naturally occurring chemicals can be toxic.
(4) Although testing studies are designed to predict adverse effects to humans, every test system has its limitations which complicate any conclusions being made about the relevance of test results to human hazard.

There are several reasons for the intense interest in developing alternative testing methods. Firstly, several types of animal test are time-consuming and costly, especially those for detection of cancer-causing chemicals. This means that there are limitations to the numbers of chemicals that can be tested. Secondly, as mentioned above, even the use of animals cannot provide definitive proof of safety or hazard. Thirdly, it is desirable from a humane point of view to reduce the numbers of animals used. However, it is only too apparent at the present time that it is impossible to eliminate the use of animals altogether if society wishes to be aware of toxic hazards.

The introduction of other testing methods has, nevertheless, begun to reduce the proportion of animals used. A large number of different tests have been developed. Generally they involve observations of the induction of toxic changes to either organisms other than man and mammals, or to parts of organisms which have been removed from animals or humans. The first example includes organisms as diverse as viruses, fruit flies and sea urchins. The second category comprises studies with cells (the individual components of organisms) which are grown free of the body, or organs such as the intestine and liver which can be maintained outside the body for short periods of time. Many alternative assays rely on the fact that the body is made up of thousands of individual units called cells. Although these vary in their appearance and roles, they all share many fundamental features with each other and with cells of widely differing organisms. Therefore many toxic effects can be studied at the cellular level.

A complication in the development of these tests is that humans, as well as other animals, possess the means for altering the structure and therefore the properties of chemicals once they are inside the body. The reason for this is that chemicals, especially many toxic substances which are not meant to be present as part of the makeup of organisms, have to be excreted to avoid their building up inside. This is a process known as detoxification. It is carried out by many different enzymes (molecules which cause the many chemical reactions of metabolism to occur).

Unfortunately, during detoxification, which is a complicated sequence of steps, chemicals can be changed into more dangerous, reactive forms which can remain in the body long enough to cause toxic changes. Therefore a chemical which is itself non-toxic outside the body can be altered inside so that it becomes toxic. This is called activation.

Altered chemicals are excreted mainly in urine by the kidneys. Therefore if these organs are unable to work properly, either because of a defect or as a consequence of damage, detoxification in general will be less good. The efficiency and way chemicals are dealt with, absorbed, activated, detoxified and excreted can differ according to the type of animal, the organ or tissue within the same animal and the age of the organism. This is why, in the past, certain additives have not been allowed for foods intended for babies and young children and why, in its latest report, the FAC has suggested that there should be an even greater restriction on the addition of colourings to such foods.

It is also the reason why certain tissues in the body are more sensitive to injury than others, and why particular species and individuals of the same species vary in their susceptibilies to the same substance. An example of this is the need for people who suffer from 'aspirin-sensitivity' to avoid certain food additives. This can be due to a genetic defect which results in the non-functioning of an enzyme called glucose-6-phosphate dehydrogenase. This enzyme is necessary to protect the haemoglobin in our red corpuscles from being oxidized by something other than oxygen. Haemoglobin is the protein responsible for transporting the oxygen inhaled to all the body cells. If it is oxidized by another chemical, obviously it will not be able to carry oxygen. Several food additives can affect haemoglobin in this way and therefore they are more likely to cause anaemia in individuals carrying this deficiency. A more direct cause of anaemia by aspirin and other chemicals is due to their rapid conversion in the intestines of some people to acids. This results in internal bleeding.

The liver is the main organ in the body where detoxification (and therefore activation) of chemicals occurs. Thus anybody with a damaged liver will have a lower capacity for detoxification. Several additives are known to cause liver damage. With respect to dietary constituents like additives it should not be forgotten that the intestinal wall itself is also a site of metabolism. Some additives can increase the amount of liver enzyme activity. If detoxification is promoted, then such an additive will increase the body's ability to excrete this and other chemicals in an innocuous form. On the other hand, activation may now occur more readily.

Obviously a chemical which is absorbed efficiently from the intestine is more likely to be toxic than one that is absorbed to a lesser extent. Generally, additives are absorbed fairly readily. Nevertheless, low absorption cannot be taken automatically as evidence of safety since the intestinal wall is still exposed and is a potential site for tumour formation and injury (for example ulceration, colitis). Damage here could affect absorption of food. Therefore it is clear that the extent to which an additive is stored in the body depends on many factors.

Activation of chemicals is known to occur, without the need for enzymes, by a chemical process called nitrosation. This involves the production of very reactive chemicals called nitrosamines. Nitrosamines are associated with several forms of toxicity including human stomach cancer. They arise by the interaction of some naturally occurring food constituents with nitrite, which is found in several food additives. It is perhaps ironic that one of the major sources of nitrite in the body is provided by nitrates in vegetables. These are converted into nitrites by bacteria in the mouth and intestine.

Two examples of alternative test methods are the Ames test which uses bacteria to detect chemicals causing inherited changes and cancer, and the use of cells outside the body in tissue culture for determining sensitization and the ability to produce skin irritation. Tissue cultures are used for many different effects, especially for detection of injury to chromosomes. The justification for using each particular short-term assay is based upon a validation procedure. This involves establishing an experimental relationship between chemical activity as detected in the assay and as seen in the intact animal or in humans exposed to the chemical. However, such a relationship is by no means perfect. Thus, for example, many chemicals which cause a mutagenic effect on the Ames assay are also known to be capable of producing tumours in man or in experimental animals (i.e. they act as both mutagens and carcinogens respectively). However, not all carcinogens turn out to be mutagens and vice versa.

In the case of sensitization there is a large amount of evidence suggesting a relationship between ability to cause irritation in the eyes of rabbits and the efficiency with which cells in culture are killed by a test chemical. Once again, though, this relationship does not hold always. Also it is not possible in most cases to predict from the results of such tests whether or not a chemical will exert a strong, intermediate or weak effect in man.

It should be added that the development of short-term assays for toxicity usually derives from a scientific basis. For example, most tests for carcinogens involve looking for DNA damage because this is known to be the initial change that occurs in cells which eventually grow into tumours. Similarly, during irritation and sensitization of tissue, changes occur in cells which can result in cell death.

Quite often the reasons for these discrepancies are understood. For example, they may be due to the fact that bacterial cells differ in certain respects in their structure and function from human cells or because the chemical is directly in contact with cells outside rather than inside the body. Nevertheless, in many cases explanations for such divergent activities are still being sought.

There are several toxic effects, such as sterility (reproductive function) which are very difficult or impossible to study without using whole animals. Alternative assays often are more sensitive than tests with whole animals. For example, an additive used in foods on the basis of observed non-carcinogenicity in an animal lifetime cancer test subsequently was found to be active in the Ames test. Further, more extensive animal assays established its carcinogenicity whereupon the chemical was banned. Of many substances found to be non-carcinogenic in recent, stringent animal tests, a large proportion exhibit some sort of activity in alternative tests designed to discriminate between carcinogens and non-carcinogens.

It has been appreciated for a long time that very small alterations in molecular arrangement of certain substances can change toxicity into non-toxicity and vice versa. Sometimes the same modifications in molecular structure alter activity in these assays and sometimes they do not. Short-term assays are very useful for studying these problems and for detecting the presence of active contaminants, even at very low amounts in preparations of additives. These contaminants are present sometimes in samples certified for use in foods and it may be possible for manufacturers to eliminate them during production.

It is clear, therefore, that the results from short-term tests can erroneously forecast inactivity or activity respectively, giving rise to false negative and positive predictions. Toxicologists are therefore in a dilemma. They have large amounts of information on the activities of many chemicals in numerous tests. However, their ability to say what exactly these results mean in terms of human hazard is severely limited at the present time.

There seems to be general agreement for a tier system approach for screening chemicals for toxicity. It is suggested that initially testing should be carried out using several different short-term assays selected to detect specific types of toxicity. If activity is detected at this stage then a decision can be made as to the importance of the chemical being assessed, for example, a safer alternative could be sought to replace it. If not, then the substance should be tested further in assays including whole animal tests. If no activity is seen at this stage, then it is common practice to assume safety. As many chemicals are active at stage I of the tier system, screening tests can reduce significantly the numbers of animals used. Indeed, gradually it is becoming possible by computer analysis of many results from testing to predict the toxicities of new chemicals without actually subjecting them to any experimentation.

Regulatory authorities place much more emphasis at present on the results of animal assays. Thus, several additives cause mutations in bacteria. However, since they are unable apparently to give rise to tumours in animals, they are still permitted in foods. Unfortunately there is no widely-used test for the induction in animals of inherited mutations, passed on from generation to generation. It is conceivable therefore that this form of hazard is being overlooked. On the other hand, anything that shows an adverse effect with animals is normally not considered to be safe with respect to the particular form of toxicity under study. Whether or not the chemical is banned from use depends upon its intended usage and the type of toxicity detected. For example, with additives, authorities consider that evidence of ability to cause tumours in animals is sufficient to ban the use of the compound in food. A chemical shown to cause defects in the new born would not be permitted for use in situations where pregnant mothers can be exposed.

Food additives comprise a group of extremely diverse chemicals which are added intentionally to many different types of food. Normally they have neither a nutritive function nor any benefit after food has been eaten. However, they are used to improve visual appearance (colourants or dyes), to enhance or provide taste (flavourings), to stabilize and improve texture (e.g. antioxidants) and to inhibit spoilage (preservatives). With modern methods of food production, storage and dispersal, additives are often necessary since food can deteriorate in one or more of these properties. In other instances the use of additives provides the food industry with alternative, more efficient and cheaper ways of processing food.

Additives are often thought of as being either 'artificial', 'natural' or 'nature-identical'. Both 'artificial' and 'nature-identical' additives are man-made in the laboratory. 'Natural' additives, on the other hand, are obtained directly from plants and animals. Currently there is a tendency for manufacturers to replace 'artificial' additives with either 'nature-identical' or 'natural' alternatives. Indeed it is common to see labels proclaiming that the food is free of all 'artificial' additives. It should not be assumed that this practice will necessarily improve the safety of the food since both 'natural' and 'nature-identical' additives can for several reasons be toxic. Firstly, as mentioned earlier, not all chemicals normally present in living organisms are harmless. Secondly, commercial preparations of these types of additives may contain harmful contaminants in the form of by-products and excess solvents used in the isolation. More research needs to be done before the replacement of 'artificial' additives in this way can be considered beneficial.

The use of food additives poses different risk-benefit problems. On the one hand colourings like Brown FK (154) are used. These are purely cosmetic and this contrasts with the use of, for example, the preservative sodium nitrite. This is added to avoid the presence of a very dangerous bacterial toxin (poisonous chemical) in certain foods. Testing has shown that both these additives may be toxic to man. Brown FK is used to satisfy an alleged consumer demand for kippered herrings with a smoked appearance, and manufacturers prefer to add the colour in order to reduce or eliminate smoking. This simplifies food production and the smoking process itself produces several toxic chemicals. Therefore the use of the colour may reduce toxicity overall. However, this depends upon the relative activities and types of effects caused by the colour and the products of smoking. At the present time this problem cannot be resolved.

Food additives are an example of a group of chemicals given priority toxicity testing since they are ingested directly, often on a regular basis over long periods of time. Usually they are present in small amounts in food and are taken into the body in combination with many other additives and food constituents which can alter their activity. Additives also can undergo changes due to food processing, cooking and preparation. Very little attention has been paid to these factors in testing them for toxicity. Thus they are tested usually at much higher concentrations than those encountered during normal exposure. However, the feeding of additives to experimental animals is not always carried out for long periods, and this may compensate to some extent for the high concentrations used.

It is customary to calculate the 'acceptable daily intake' (A.D.I.) for each additive. This is done by taking the maximum amount of chemical shown to produce no toxic effect after feeding to a test animal (the no effect level or N.E.L.). This value is then divided by a number representing a safety factor which is used to guard against the possibility that the toxicity tests undertaken to establish the N.E.L. were too insensitive. The value of this number can vary, but is usually 100. Under certain circumstances 'temporary A.D.I.' values are issued by regulatory authorities, especially when more toxicological information is required. The idea is that the levels of an additive present in foods should be such that the A.D.I. value for each is not exceeded. This does not take into account that, collectively, the A.D.I. values for a group of additives might be greater than the A.D.I. for any one of them when foods containing mixtures of additives are consumed.

Recently there has been much public concern over the possible relationship between behaviour and the intake of certain food additives. There have been many documented cases of intolerance and hyperactivity, especially in children. These reports have been widespread, geographically, and have been linked to the presence of these additives in food previously consumed. Unfortunately, much of this evidence has been anecdotal and there has been some reluctance on the part of regulatory bodies and manufacturers to respond until detailed experimental verification of this association is forthcoming. In the past, there have been several attempts, using clinical trials under controlled conditions, to demonstrate effects on behaviour caused by intake of food containing certain additives. Also additive-free diets have been prepared and used to alleviate symptoms of hyperactivity. The results of all these studies to date are inconclusive. However, it is clear that several experiments, claiming no effect of additives, were incorrectly carried out. Moreover, it is known that some additives implicated in hyperactivity can cause allergies and sensitization in man, and can affect nerve function and be transported to brain cells in experimental animals, under certain circumstances. So the problem of hyperactivity deserves further investigation to determine whether or not there is a scientific basis for additive-induced hyperactivity. In the meantime, it can be concluded that there is sufficient evidence to suggest that certain children do exhibit disturbed behaviour after consuming food containing particular additives. The result of some trials, currently in progress, should help to establish the extent of this phenomenon.

Appendix II
Warning:
Dangerous Food Additives
The Villejuif List

E for Additives was certainly a bestseller, but the distribution of the fraudulent Villejuif list must make the number of copies of *E for Additives* sold look insignificant.

The list came to prominence without the E numbers some eight or nine years ago and a quick check with the two hospitals mentioned, Villejuif and Chaumont, drew instant denials that they had anything to do with it. The French, Belgian and British governments have all issued statements pointing out that it was a forgery.

Yet, with distressing frequency, we find people saying that they follow the advice in *E for Additives* but have a very useful list from the Villejuif Hospital which summarizes it! The author even burnt a copy of the list in public on the BBC Television 'Food and Drink Programme' and, as a result, some groups distributing it have now taken a more responsible attitude and have either modified or discontinued the text.

The sad fact is that this inaccurate information about additives has been distributed by kind, good and certainly well-meaning people who sincerely believe they are helping others. Nothing could be farther from the truth. See the photograph of the Villejuif list on page 306. If you turn to the entry in this book for E330, citric acid, you will see how this harmless substance gained a false reputation for being one of the most dangerous of all additives. The difficulty is that there are a number of half-truths within the list, and we think it is a useful exercise to go through the various adverse statements and form your own conclusions by making comparisons with the reviews of each additive in this book.

The use of additives cannot normally be considered by using a 'traffic light' system of good, suspicious and dangerous because

WARNING: DANGEROUS FOOD ADDITIVES

This is a list of the food colourings and additives that has been prepared by the
Hospital Centre of Chaumont, France, based on information given by the Research Centre
Hospital of Villejuif, France, to draw the attention of all consumers to the effects of
additives used in the food industry.

E100	Harmless	E230	Skin Disturbance
E101	Harmless	E231	Skin Disturbance
E102	Dangerous	E232	Skin Disturbance
E103	Forbidden	E233	Skin Disturbance
E104	Suspicious	E236	Harmless
E105	Forbidden	E237	Harmless
E110	Dangerous	E238	Harmless
E111	Forbidden	E239	Carcinogenic Product
E120	Dangerous	E240	Suspicious
E121	Forbidden	E241	Suspicious
E122	Suspicious	E250	Blood Pressure Incident
E123	Very Dangerous (Monster Munch)	E251	Blood Pressure Incident
E124	Dangerous	E252	Blood Pressure Incident
E125	Forbidden	E260	Harmless
E126	Forbidden	E261	Harmless
E127	Dangerous	E262	Harmless
E130	Forbidden	E263	Harmless
E131	Carcinogenic Product	E270	Harmless
E132	Harmless	E280	Harmless
E140	Harmless	E281	Harmless
E141	Suspicious	E282	Harmless
E142	Carcinogenic Product	E300	Harmless
E150	Suspicious	E301	Harmless
E151	Suspicious	E302	Harmless
E152	Forbidden	E303	Harmless
E153	Suspicious	E304	Harmless
E160	Harmless	E305	Harmless
E161	Harmless	E306	Harmless
E163	Harmless	E307	Harmless
E170	Harmless	E308	Harmless
E171	Suspicious	E309	Harmless
E173	Suspicious	E311	Skin Rash
E174	Harmless	E312	Skin Rash
E175	Harmless	E320	Cholesterol)
E180	Suspicious	E321	Cholesterol) Crisps
E181	Forbidden	E322	Harmless
E200	Harmless	E325	Harmless
E201	Harmless	E326	Harmless
E202	Harmless	E327	Harmless
E203	Harmless	E330	Carcinogenic Product & Cold Sores
E210	Carcinogenic Product	E331	Harmless
E211	Carcinogenic Product	E332	Harmless
E212	Carcinogenic Product	E333	Harmless
E213	Carcinogenic Product	E334	Harmless
E214	Carcinogenic Product	E335	Harmless
E215	Carcinogenic Product	E336	Harmless
E217	Carcinogenic Product	E337	Harmless
E220	Destruction of Vitamin B12	E338	Digestive Disturbance
E221	Intestinal Disturbance	E339	Digestive Disturbance
E223	Intestinal Disturbance	E340	Digestive Disturbance
E224	Intestinal Disturbance	E341	Digestive Disturbance
E226	Intestinal Disturbance	E400	Harmless

/over

E401	Harmless		E422	Harmless
E402	Harmless		E450	Digestive Disturbance
E403	Harmless		E461	Digestive Disturbance
E404	Harmless		E462	Digestive Disturbance
E406	Harmless		E463	Digestive Disturbance
E407	Digestive Disturbance		E465	Digestive Disturbance
E408	Harmless		E466	Digestive Disturbance
E410	Harmless		E471	Harmless
E411	Harmless		E472	Harmless
E413	Harmless		E473	Harmless
E414	Harmless		E474	Harmless
E420	Harmless		E475	Harmless
E421	Harmless		E477	Suspicious

Explanatory Notes:

Carcinogenic - Substance which can cause cancerous cells to form.

Forbidden - Forbidden by the French Health Minister 1st January 1977

Harmless - Harmless Substances

Suspicious - Suspicious products with side effects currently under study.

Destruction of Vitamin B12 - Destroys Vitamin B12 which is vital for proper
functioning of the nervous system.

Blood Pressure Incidents - Present in pre-cooked meats.

E123 - Very dangerous, has been prohibited in the USSR and USA.

All of these additives are presently permitted in Britain and are shown on food
packings. RESTRAIN the abusive use of these additives by chosing the products that
you are buying. Remember, it is the consumer who decides and imposes the options of
the food manufacturers. Think of your childrens' health. Reproduce this document,
distribute it around and, use it. Your health is your life.

the issues involved are much more complicated than that. We do believe, however, that certain additives are either unnecessary or that their possible risks outweigh any benefits.

Toxicity is linked to dosage. You can die from drinking a vast quantity of water or from just 100g of common salt, yet in the right quantities both these substances are important to health. So, campaign with your friends for the rejection of the Villejuif list and resolve to make your own selection of any additives which you would rather do without.

Appendix III
The Regulation of Food Additives

The Food Advisory Committee (FAC) approved food additives in a complex and potentially efficient way.

The Ministry of Food makes it clear that the members of the FAC do not sign the Official Secrets Act but that nevertheless they cannot disclose information which has been given them for specific purposes by officials or commercial companies. In practice this means that, when compiling books like this where we try to take a balanced and non-biased view, we are severely limited because so much of the positive evidence for certain additives and, no doubt, the negative also, is not for our eyes. The Freedom of Information regulations in the USA are in direct contrast, and so certain of our research material has come from the United States and other sources which are not available to the general public.

Now there are definite difficulties even in persuading people to publish so much specialist research. The Ministry has now arranged that, in future, copies of toxicological data considered during reviews by the FAC will be available at the British Library. This is a positive and helpful move but does not get us a whole way along the road towards evaluating again those many additives that have already gone through the mill.

Let us look at the flow chart for the consideration of food additives (see pages 310 and 311).

All these well-meaning and dedicated people are certainly trying to do a good job for us humble eaters, but they can have very different values from us. Most important is the definition of need.

As the Ministry says, the general principle which accepts an additive says that it is permitted in food only where:

(1) there is a genuine demonstrable need;
(2) it can be established to the satisfaction of the Committee on Toxicity of Chemicals in Food, Consumer Products and the Environment (COT) that its use would not prejudice the health of consumers;
(3) there is satisfactory evidence that its presence would not adversely affect the nutritive value of food;
(4) it conforms with an adequate and appropriate specification of purity.

Furthermore:

(5) the quantity of any additive permitted in food should, where necessary, be restricted to that which in the judgement of the Committee is needed to achieve its effect; and
(6) the addition of any additive to a food should be identified to the consumer to enable an informed choice to be made.

Assessment of 'Need'

In assessing the need for a particular additive the FAC must be satisfied by adequate supporting evidence that there is a clear benefit to the consumer that cannot reasonably be achieved by use of an already permitted additive, or by any other means. In deciding whether there is benefit to the consumer, the Committee will take into account:

(1) the need to maintain the wholesomeness of food products up to the time they are consumed;
(2) the need for food to be presented in a palatable and attractive manner;
(3) convenience in purchasing, packaging, storage, preparation, and use;
(4) the extension of dietary choice;
(5) the need for nutritional supplementation; and
(6) any economic advantage.

Labelling

The Committee will also consider and recommend any labelling

Ministry of Agriculture, Fisheries and Food
FLOW CHART FOR CONSIDERATION OF FOOD ADDITIVES

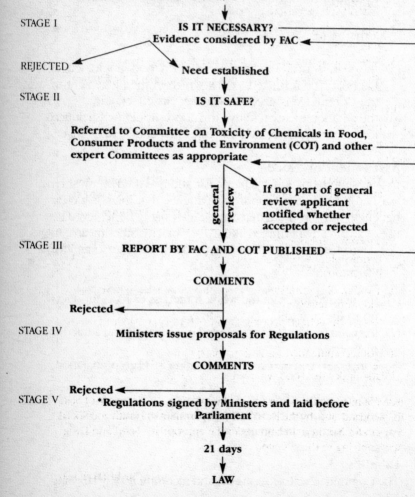

AN ADDITIVE

↓

Referred by the Minister of Agriculture, Fisheries and
Food, the Secretaries of State for Social Services, Wales
and Scotland and the Head of the Department of Health
and Social Services for Northern Ireland to the FOOD
ADVISORY COMMITTEE (FAC)

↓

STAGE I — **IS IT NECESSARY?**
Evidence considered by FAC ◄

REJECTED ◄ — **Need established**

STAGE II — **IS IT SAFE?**

↓

Referred to Committee on Toxicity of Chemicals in Food,
Consumer Products and the Environment (COT) and other
expert Committees as appropriate ◄

general review

**If not part of general
review applicant
notified whether
accepted or rejected**

STAGE III — **REPORT BY FAC AND COT PUBLISHED** —

COMMENTS

Rejected ◄

STAGE IV — **Ministers issue proposals for Regulations**

COMMENTS

Rejected ◄
STAGE V — ***Regulations signed by Ministers and laid before
Parliament**

21 days

↓

LAW

REASONS FOR REFERRAL

Because

1. General review of that particular class of additive.
2. Consideration of a further group of additives.
3. A firm wants (a) a new additive or (b) an extension of the conditions of use imposed on a currently permitted additive.

EXAMPLES OF NEED FOR AN ADDITIVE

1. Required in manufacturing process. Other permitted additives or food substances are not suitable.
2. Improved product for consumer (e.g. improved taste or appearance).
3. New product requiring additive use not presently permitted.
4. An economic need (e.g. cheaper product, longer shelf life).

Evidence considered

1. Industry's or firm's own or sponsored research.
2. Research by BIBRA or other research association.
3. Any work in related field — published or unpublished.
4. WHO/FAO Expert Committee on Food Additives recommendations, and EC Scientific Committee for Food recommendations.
5. Recommendations by other international organizations.

FAC recommendations:

1. Permissible — level(s) or usage and food(s) in which to be used if appropriate.
2. Temporarily permissible — as (1), plus an indication of when it should be reviewed.
3. Not recommended pending supply of further evidence of need or safety.
4. Not recommended for and reason(s) why.

*Made under the Food Act 1984.

Note: Similar regulations are normally made by the Secretary of State for Scotland and by the Head of the Department of Health and Social Services for Northern Ireland under the appropriate Food and Drugs Acts applying to those countries.

Standards Division

provisions that may be necessary to ensure that the consumer is not misled as to the nature, substance or quality of the food to which an additive may be added.

My old friend Cyril Scott said to me when in his nineties, after offering me a cream-filled meringue for tea, that having some of the enjoyable and fun foods in life is no problem to a healthy person, provided he takes enough of the right foods. The 'E' number code helps us to decide upon our own balance and remember that very many additives are used as good and necessary parts of a modern diet.

The following is the list of the main regulations applying to food additives:

SI Number

1978 No. 105   *The Antioxidants in Food Regulations 1978* as amended by

1980 No. 1831 *The Antioxidants in Food (Amendment) Regulations 1980,*

1983 No. 1211 *The Sweeteners in Food Regulations 1983*, and

1984 No. 1304 *The Bread and Flour Regulations 1984,*

lay down a list of permitted antioxidants and specifications of purity for each substance; for certain antioxidants, specify the foods in which they may be used and the maximum levels of use; prescribe labelling requirements for antioxidants sold as such, and prohibit the sale of foods described as intended for babies or young children containing certain antioxidants.

1980 No. 36   *The Chloroform in Food Regulations 1980,* make it an offence to sell or import food containing added chloroform.

1973 No. 1340 *The Colouring Matter in Food Regulations 1973,* as amended by

1974 No. 1119 *The Preservatives in Food Regulations 1974,*

1975 No. 1488 *The Colouring Matter in Food (Amendment) Regulations 1975,*

1976 No. 2086 *The Colouring Matter in Food (Amendment) Regulations 1976,* and

1978 No. 1787 *The Colouring Matter in Food (Amendment) Regulations 1978,*
lay down a list of permitted colouring matter and specifications of purity for each substance; for certain colours specify the foods in which they may be used and prescribe labelling requirements for colours sold as such.

1980 No. 1833 *The Emulsifiers and Stabilizers in Food Regulations 1980* as amended by

1982 No. 16 *The Emulsifiers and Stabilizers in Food (Amendment) Regulations 1982,*

1983 No. 1211 *The Sweeteners in Food Regulations 1983,*

1983 No. 1810 *The Emulsifiers and Stabilizers in Food (Amendment) Regulations 1983,*

1984 No. 649 *The Cheese (Amendment) Regulations 1984,* and

1984 No. 1304 *The Bread and Flour Regulations 1984,*
lay down a list of permitted emulsifiers and permitted stabilizers and specifications of purity for each substance; for certain emulsifiers and stabilizers specify the food in which they may be used and maximum levels of use; list certain foods in which the use of permitted emulsifiers and stabilizers is limited and prescribe labelling requirements for emulsifiers and stabilizers sold as such.

1964 No. 19 *The Meat (Treatment) Regulations 1964*
prohibit the use of any raw and unprocessed meat intended for sale for human consumption of any added substance specified in the Regulations.

1966 No. 1073 *The Mineral Hydrocarbons in Food Regulations 1966* prohibit (subject to certain exceptions relating to dried fruits, citrus fruits, sugar confectionery, lubricants, the rind of cheese, eggs and chewing compounds) the use of any mineral hydrocarbon in the composition or preparation of food; lay down specifications for mineral hydrocarbons and the method of testing solid mineral hydrocarbons for the presence of polycyclic hydrocarbon.

1980 No. 1834 *The Miscellaneous Additives in Food Regulations 1980* as amended by

1980 No. 1849 *The Food Labelling Regulations 1980*,

1982 No. 14 The Miscellaneous Additives in Food (Amendment) Regulations 1982,

1983 No. 1211 *The Sweeteners in Food Regulations 1983*, and

1984 No. 1304 *The Bread and Flour Regulations 1984*, control by permitted list fifteen classes of food additives; provide specifications of purity for each substance; for certain miscellaneous additives specify the foods in which they may be used and prescribe labelling requirements for miscellaneous additives sold as such. The classes are: acids, anti-caking and anti-foaming agents, bases, buffers, firming and glazing agents, humectants, liquid freezants, packaging gases, propellants, release agents, sequestrants, bulking aids and flavour modifiers.

1979 No. 752 *The Preservatives in Food Regulations 1979* as amended by

1980 No. 931 *The Preservatives in Food (Amendment) Regulations 1980*,

1981 No. 1063 *The Jam and Similar Products Regulations 1981*,

1982 No. 15 *The Preservatives in Food (Amendment) Regulations 1982*,

1982 No. 1311 *The Fruit Juices and Fruit Nectars (Amendment) Regulations 1982*,

1983 No. 1211   *The Sweeteners in Food Regulations 1983*, and

1984 No. 1304   *The Bread and Flour Regulations 1984*,

lay down a list of permitted preservatives and specifications of purity for each substance; specify the foods in which they may be used and maximum levels of use, and prescribe labelling requirements for preservatives sold as such.

1967 No. 1582   *The Solvents in Food Regulations 1967*, as amended by

1967 No. 1939   *The Solvents in Food (Amendment) Regulations 1967*,

1980 No. 1832   *The Solvents in Food (Amendment) Regulations 1980*,

1983 No. 1211   *The Sweeteners in Food Regulations 1983*, and

1984 No. 1304   *The Bread and Flour Regulations 1984*,

lay down a list of permitted carrier solvents and specifications of purity for each substance and prescribe labelling requirements for solvents sold as such.

1983 No. 1211   *The Sweeteners in Food Regulations 1983*

lay down a list of permitted sweeteners and specifications of purity for each substance, and prescribe labelling requirements for sweeteners sold as such where not already covered by the *Food Labelling Regulations 1980* (as amended).

1987   *The Consumer Protection Act 1987*.

A Manufacturer has no liability under the Act if approved additives up to such limits as may be imposed by The Food Act 1984 adversely affect a consumer. If, however, there are no statutory limits and the additive is used to excess, there could be liability.

1984 No. 1305   *The Food Labelling Regulations 1984*

set out labelling requirements, durability,

instructions, indication of additives, alcoholic drinks, claims and misleading descriptions.

1984   *The Food Act 1984.*
        The basic legal framework which provides the foundation upon which fod regulations are made and interpreted.

Alphabetical List of Additives and Their E Numbers

E414	Acacia
E260	Acetic acid
E472(a)	Acetic acid esters of mono- and di-glycerides of fatty acids
E142	Acid Brilliant Green
E341(a)	Acid calcium phosphate
E450(a)	Acid sodium pyrophosphate
355	Adipic acid
E406	Agar
621	Aji-no-moto
E405	Alginate ester
E400	Alginic acid
E160(a)	Alpha-carotene
E460	Alpha-cellulose
E173	Aluminium
556	Aluminium calcium silicate
559	Aluminium silicate
554	Aluminium sodium silicate
E123	Amaranth
E440(b)	Amidated pectin
E403	Ammonium alginate
503	Ammonium carbonate
510	Ammonium chloride
381	Ammonium ferric citrate
381	Ammonium ferric citrate, green
503	Ammonium hydrogen carbonate
527	Ammonium hydroxide
442	Ammonium phosphatides

545	Ammonium polyphosphates
E160(b)	Annatto
E163	Anthocyanins
E300	L-Ascorbic acid
E304	Ascorbyl palmitate
927	Azodicarbonamide
927	Azoformamide
E122	Azorubine
500	Baking soda
901	Beeswax, white
901	Beeswax, yellow
E162	Beetroot Red
558	Bentonite
E210	Benzoic acid
E160(e)	beta-apo-8'-carotenal
E162	Betanin
E320	BHA
E321	BHT
500	Bicarbonate of soda
E230	Biphenyl
E161(b)	Bixin
E151	Black PN
542	Bone phosphate
133	Brilliant blue FCF
154	Brown FK
155	Brown HT
E320	Butylated hydroxyanisole
E321	Butylated hydroxytoluene
E263	Calcium acetate
E404	Calcium alginate
E302	Calcium L-ascorbate
E213	Calcium benzoate
E227	Calcium bisulphite
E170	Calcium carbonate
509	Calcium chloride
509	Calcium chloride; anhydrous
623	Calcium dihydrogen di-L-glutamate

385	Calcium disodium EDTA
385	Calcium disodium ethylenediamine-NNN'N tetra-acetate
E238	Calcium formate
578	Calcium gluconate
623	Calcium glutamate
352	Calcium hydrogen malate
E341(b)	Calcium hydrogen orthophosphate
E227	Calcium hydrogen sulphate
526	Calcium hydroxide
E327	Calcium lactate
352	Calcium malate
529	Calcium oxide
E341(c)	Calcium phosphate tribasic
544	Calcium polyphosphates
E282	Calcium propionate
552	Calcium silicate
E203	Calcium sorbate
E482	Calcium stearoyl-2-lactylate
516	Calcium sulphate
E226	Calcium sulphite
E341(a)	Calcium tetrahydrogen diorthophosphate
E161(g)	Canthaxanthin
E160(c)	Capsanthin
E160(c)	Capsorubin
E150	Caramel
E153	Carbon black
E290	Carbon dioxide
E466	Carboxymethylcellulose, sodium salt
E120	Carmine of cochineal
E120	Carminic acid
E122	Carmoisine
903	Carnauba wax
E410	Carob gum
E160(a)	Carotene, alpha-, beta- and gamma-

E407	Carrageenan
524	Caustic soda
E465	Cellulose, ethyl methyl
E463	Cellulose hydroxypropyl
E464	Cellulose hydroxypropylmethyl
E460(i)	Cellulose, microcrystalline
E460(ii)	Cellulose, powdered
925	Chlorine
926	Chlorine dioxide
E140	Chlorophyll
154	Chocolate brown FK
155	Chocolate brown HT
E330	Citric acid
E472(c)	Citric acid esters of mono- and di-glycerides of fatty acids
380	Citric acid triammonium salt
E472(c)	Citroglycerides
E466	CMC
E120	Cochineal
E124	Cochineal Red A
E461	Cologel
E336	Cream of tartar
E161(c)	Cryptoxanthin
E100	Curcumin
920	L-cysteine hydrochloride
920	L-cysteine hydrochloride monohydrate
E472(e)	Diacetyltartaric acid esters of fatty acids
E333	*di*Calcium citrate
540	*di*Calcium diphosphate
540	*di*Calcium pyrophosphate
900	Dimethicone
900	Dimethylpolysiloxane
E230	Diphenyl
E340(b)	*di*Potassium hydrogen orthophosphate
E336	*di*Potassium L-(+)-tartrate

E450(a)	*di*Sodium dihydrogen diphosphate
E339(a)	*di*Sodium hydrogen orthophosphate
E335	*di*Sodium L-(+)-tartrate
E312	Dodecyl gallate
542	Edible bone phosphate
442	Emulsifier YN
518	Epsom salts
E127	Erythrosine
E160(f)	Ethyl ester of beta-apo-8'-carotenoic acid
E214	Ethyl-4-hydroxybenzoate
E214	Ethyl para-hydroxybenzoate
E215	Ethyl-4-hydroxybenzoate, sodium salt
637	Ethyl maltol
E465	Ethylmethylcellulose
E306	Extracts of natural origin rich in tocopherols
E133	FD and C Blue 1
E132	FD and C Blue 2
E123	FD and C Red 2
E127	FD and C Red 3
E102	FD and C Yellow 5
E110	FD and C Yellow 6
381	Ferric ammonium citrate
E161(a)	Flavoxanthin
E236	Formic acid
553(b)	French chalk
297	Fumaric acid
E160(a)	Gamma-carotene
575	Glucono delta-lactone
575	D-Glucono-1,5-lactone
620	L-glutamic acid
E422	Glycerin
E422	Glycerol
E471	Glyceryl monostearate
E197	Gold
E142	Green S
627	Guanosine 5'-(*di*Sodium phosphate)

E412	Guar gum
E414	Gum arabic
370	1,4-Heptonolactone
E239	Hexamine
E239	Hexamethylenetetramine
507	Hydrochloric acid
E231	2-Hydroxybiphenyl
E463	Hydroxypropylcellulose
E464	Hydroxypropylmethylcellulose
E464	Hypromellose
E132	Indigo carmine
631	Inosine 5'-(disodium phosphate)
E172	Iron hydroxides
E172	Iron oxides
E406	Japanese isinglass
559	Kaolin
416	Karaya gum
154	Kipper Brown
E270	Lactic acid
E472(b)	Lactic acid esters of mono- and di-glycerides of fatty acids
E101	Lactoflavin
E472(b)	Lactoglycerides
478	Lactylated fatty acid esters of glycerol and propane-1,2-diol
E322	Lecithin
620	L-glutamic acid
E142	Lissamine Green
E180	Lithol Rubine BK
E410	Locust bean gum
E161(b)	Lutein
E160(d)	Lycopene
504	Magnesium carbonate
528	Magnesium hydroxide
530	Magnesium oxide
553(a)	Magnesium silicate synthetic
572	Magnesium stearate
518	Magnesium sulphate

553(a)	Magnesium trisilicate
296	DL-Malic acid, L-Malic acid
636	Maltol
E163	Malvidin
E421	Mannitol
353	Metatartaric acid
E236	Methanoic acid
E461	Methocel
E461	Methylcellulose
E218	Methyl 4-hydroxybenzoate
E218	Methyl para-hydroxybenzoate
E219	Methyl 4-hydroxybenzoate, sodium salt
E460(i)	Microcrystalline cellulose
907	Microcrystalline wax, refined
905	Mineral hydrocarbons
E472(e)	Mono- and diacetyltartaric acid esters of mono- and di-glycerides of fatty acids
E471	Mono- and di-glycerides of fatty acids
E333	*mono*Calcium citrate
E341(a)	*mono*Calcium orthophosphate
E332	*mono*Potassium citrate
622	*mono*Potassium glutamate
E336	*mono*Potassium L-(+)-tartrate
E331	*mono*Sodium citrate
621	*mono*Sodium glutamate
E335	*mono*sodium L-(+)-tartrate
621	MSG
375	Niacin
375	Nicotinic acid
234	Nisin
E160(b)	Norbixin
570	Octadecanoic acid
E311	Octyl gallate
E231	Orthophenylphenol
E338	Orthophosphoric acid

E304	6-0-Palmitoyl-L-ascorbic acid
E131	Patent blue V
E440(a)	Pectin
E163	Pelargonidin
E450(b)	*penta*Potassium triphosphate
E450(b)	*penta*Sodium triphosphate
E163	Peonidin
E163	Petunidin
E338	Phosphoric acid
E180	Pigment Rubine
E475	Polyglycerol esters of fatty acids
476	Polyglycerol esters of polycondensed fatty acids of castor oil
476	Polyglycerol polyricinoleate
432	Polyoxyethylene (20) sorbitan monolaurate
433	Polyoxyethylene (20) sorbitan mono-oleate
434	Polyoxyethylene (20) sorbitan monopalmitate
435	Polyoxyethylene (20) sorbitan monostearate
436	Polyoxyethylene (20) sorbitan tristearate
430	Polyoxyethylene (8) stearate
431	Polyoxyethylene (40) stearate
544	Polyphosphates, calcium
545	Polyphosphates, ammonium
E450(c)	Polyphosphates, potassium and sodium
432	Polysorbate 20
434	Polysorbate 40
435	Polysorbate 60
436	Polysorbate 65
433	Polysorbate 80
E124	Ponceau 4R
E261	Potassium acetate
E402	Potassium alginate

E212	Potassium benzoate
924	Potassium bromate
501	Potassium carbonate
508	Potassium chloride
E332	Potassium citrate
E332	Potassium dihydrogen citrate
E340(a)	Potassium dihydrogen orthophosphate
536	Potassium ferrocyanide
577	Potassium gluconate
536	Potassium hexacyanoferrate (II)
501	Potassium hydrogen carbonate
622	Potassium hydrogen L-glutamate
E336	Potassium hydrogen tartrate
525	Potassium hydroxide
E326	Potassium lactate
351	Potassium malate
E224	Potassium metabisulphite
E252	Potassium nitrate
E249	Potassium nitrite
E340	Potassium phosphate dibasic
E340(c)	Potassium phosphate tribasic
E402	Potassium polymannuronate
E450(c)	Potassium polyphosphates
E283	Potassium propionate
E224	Potassium pyrosulphite
E470	Potassium salts of fatty acids
E337	Potassium sodium DL-tartrate
E337	Potassium sodium L-(+)-tartrate
E202	Potassium sorbate
515	Potassium sulphate
E450(b)	Potassium tripolyphosphate
E460(ii)	Powdered cellulose
E405	Propane -1, 1-diol alginate
E477	Propane -1, 2-diol esters of fatty acids
E280	Propionic acid
E405	Propylene glycol alginate

E310	Propyl gallate
E216	Propyl 4-hydroxybenzoate
E216	Propyl para-hydroxybenzoate
E217	Propyl 4-hydroxybenzoate, sodium salt
529	Quicklime
E104	Quinoline yellow
128	Red 2G
907	Refined microcrystalline wax
E161(f)	Rhodoxanthin
E101	Riboflavin
101(a)	Riboflavin-5'-phosphate
E337	Rochelle salt
E160(b)	Rocou
E180	Rubine
E161(d)	Rubixanthin
E252	Saltpetre
E341(b)	Secondary calcium phosphate
904	Shellac
551	Silica
551	Silicon dioxide
E174	Silver
900	Simethicone
558	Soap clay
262	Sodium acetate
E401	Sodium alginate
554	Sodium aluminosilicate
541	Sodium aluminium phosphate
E301	Sodium L-ascorbate
E211	Sodium benzoate
500	Sodium bicarbonate
E232	Sodium biphenyl-2-yl oxide
E222	Sodium bisulphite
500	Sodium carbonate
E466	Sodium carboxymethylcellulose
E262	Sodium diacetate
E331	Sodium dihydrogen citrate
E339(a)	Sodium dihydrogen orthophosphate

E215	Sodium ethyl para-hydroxybenzoate
535	Sodium ferrocyanide
E237	Sodium formate
576	Sodium gluconate
627	Sodium guanylate
535	Sodium hexacyanoferrate (II)
500	Sodium hydrogen carbonate
E262	Sodium hydrogen diacetate
621	Sodium hydrogen L-glutamate
350	Sodium hydrogen malate
E222	Sodium hydrogen sulphite
524	Sodium hydroxide
631	Sodium inosinate
E325	Sodium lactate
350	Sodium malate
E223	Sodium metabisulphite
E219	Sodium methyl para-hydroxybenzoate
E251	Sodium nitrate
E250	Sodium nitrite
E232	Sodium orthophenylphenate
E450(c)	Sodium polyphosphates
E337	Sodium potassium tartrate
E281	Sodium propionate
E217	Sodium propyl para-hydroxybenzoate
635	Sodium 5'-ribonucleotide
E470	Sodium salts of fatty acids
500	Sodium sesquicarbonate
E201	Sodium sorbate
E481	Sodium stearoyl-2-lactylate
514	Sodium sulphate
E221	Sodium sulphite
E335	Sodium L-(+)-tartrate
E450(b)	Sodium tripolyphosphate
E200	Sorbic acid
493	Sorbitan monolaurate
494	Sorbitan mono-oleate

495	Sorbitan monopalmitate
491	Sorbitan monostearate
492	Sorbitan tristearate
E420(i)	Sorbitol
E420(ii)	Sorbitol syrup
493	Span 20
495	Span 40
492	Span 65
494	Span 80
570	Stearic acid
E483	Stearyl tartrate
363	Succinic acid
E474	Sucroglycerides
E473	Sucrose esters of fatty acids
E220	Sulphur dioxide
513	Sulphuric acid
E110	Sunset yellow FCF
E307	Synthetic alpha-tocopherol
E308	Synthetic beta-tocopherol
E309	Synthetic delta-tocopherol
553(b)	Talc
E334	L-(+)-tartaric acid
E472(d)	Tartaric acid esters of mono- and di-glycerides of fatty acids
E102	Tartrazine
E450(a)	*tetra*Potassium diphosphate
E450(a)	*tetra*Sodium diphosphate
E450(a)	*tetra*Sodium pyrophosphate
E233	Thiabendazole
E171	Titanium dioxide
E307	*alpha*-Tocopherol, synthetic
E309	*delta*-Tocopherol, synthetic
E308	*beta*-Tocopherol, synthetic
E306	Tocopherols, extracts of natural origin
E413	Tragacanth
380	*tri*Ammonium citrate

E333	*tri*Calcium citrate
E341(c)	*tri*Calcium diorthophosphate
E332	*tri*Potassium citrate
E340(c)	*tri*Potassium orthophosphate
E331	*tri*Sodium citrate
E450(a)	*tri*Sodium diphosphate
E339(c)	*tri*Sodium orthophosphate
E153	Vegetable carbon
E161(e)	Violoxanthin
375	Vitamin B complex
E101	Vitamin B$_2$
E300	Vitamin C
E306	Vitamin E (natural)
E307	Vitamin E (synthetic)
E308	Vitamin E (synthetic)
E309	Vitamin E (synthetic)
907	Wax, refined, microcrystalline
E415	Xanthan gum
E161	Xanthophylls
107	Yellow 2G

List of Categories of Food Additives

(A listing of the principal additives by function including some which have not been given numbers.)

Acidity Regulators (E260–380)

E260	Acetic acid
E261	Potassium acetate
262	Sodium acetate
E263	Calcium acetate
296	Malic acid
297	Fumaric acid
E326	Potassium lactate
E327	Calcium lactate
E330	Citric acid
E331(a)	Sodium dihydrogen citrate
E331(b)	*di*Sodium citrate
E331(c)	*tri*Sodium citrate

Acids (E270–513)

E270	Lactic acid
296	Malic acid
E334	Tartaric acid
E336	*mono*Potassium tartrate
E338	Orthophosphoric acid
363	Succinic acid
370	1,4-Heptonolactone
507	Hydrochloric acid
513	Sulphuric acid

Anti-caking Agents (E170–900)

E170	Calcium carbonate
E450(a)	*tetra*Sodium pyrophosphate
E460(i)	Microcrystalline cellulose
E460(ii)	Powdered cellulose
530	Magnesium oxide
535	Sodium hexacyanoferrate
536	Potassium hexacyanoferrate
542	Edible bone phosphate
551	Silicon dioxide
552	Calcium silicate
553(a)	Magnesium silicate (synthetic)
553(b)	Talc
554	Aluminium sodium silicate
556	Aluminium calcium silicate
558	Bentonite
559	Kaolin
570	Stearic acid
572	Magnesium stearate
900	Dimethylpolysiloxane
	Aluminium silicate
	Calcium ferrocyanide
	Calcium phosphate, tribasic
	Magnesium hydrogen carbonate
	Magnesium phosphate, tribasic
	Salts of myristic, palmitic and stearic acid with bases accepted for food use (Al, Ca, Na, Mg, K, NH_4)

Anti-foaming Agents

900	Dimethylpolysiloxane
	Oxystearin

Antioxidants (E220–E330)

E220	Sulphur dioxide
E300	L-Ascorbic acid
E301	Sodium L-ascorbate
E302	Calcium L-ascorbate

E304	Ascorbyl palmitate
E306	Extracts of natural origin rich in tocopherols
E307	Synthetic alpha-tocopherol
E308	Synthetic gamma-tocopherol
E309	Synthetic delta-tocopherol
E310	Propyl gallate
E311	Octyl gallate
E312	Dodecyl gallate
E320	Butylated hydroxyanisole
E321	Butylated hydroxytoluene
E322	Lecithins
E330	Citric acid
	Anoxomer
	Ascorbyl stearate
	Dilaury thiodipropionate
	Diphenylamine
	Distearyl thiodipropionate
	Ethoxyquin
	Ethyl protocatechuate
	Guaiac resin
	Hydroxymethyl 1-2,6-ditertiary-butylphenol (4)
	Isoamylgallate
	Isoascorbic acid
	Isopropyl citrate mixture
	Nordihydroguaiaretic acid
	Potassium ascorbate
	Sodium erythorbate
	Sodium thiosulphate
	Stannous chloride
	Tertiary butylhydroquinone
	Thiodipropionic acid

Colours (E100–E180)

E100	Curcumin
E101	Riboflavin
101(a)	Riboflavin-5'-phosphate
E102	Tartrazine
E104	Quinoline yellow

107	Yellow 2G
E110	Sunset yellow FCF
E120	Cochineal
E122	Carmoisine
E123	Amaranth
E124	Ponceau 4R
E127	Erythrosine
128	Red 2G
E131	Patent blue V
E132	Indigo carmine
133	Brilliant blue FCF
E140	Chlorophyll
E141	Copper complexes of chlorophyll and chlorophyllins
E142	Green S
E150	Caramel
E151	Black PN
E153	Carbon black (vegetable carbon)
154	Brown FK
155	Brown HT (Chocolate brown HT)
E160(a)	Alpha-carotene, beta-carotene, gamma-carotene
E160(b)	Annatto; bixin; norbixin
E160(c)	Capsanthin; capsorubin
E160(d)	Lycopene
E160(e)	Beta-apo-8'-carotenal
E160(f)	Ethyl ester of beta-apo-8'-carotenoic acid
E161(a)	Flavoxanthin
E161(b)	Lutein
E161(c)	Cryptoxanthin
E161(d)	Rubixanthin
E161(e)	Violoxanthin
E161(f)	Rhodoxanthin
E161(g)	Canthaxanthin
E162	Beetroot red (betanin)
E163	Anthocyanins
E171	Titanium dioxide
E172	Iron oxides; iron hydroxides
E173	Aluminium

E174   Silver
E175   Gold
E180   Pigment rubine
        Methyl violet
        Paprika
        Saffron
        Sandalwood
        Turmeric

Emulsifiers (E322–495)

E322   Lecithins
E400   Alginic acid
E401   Sodium alginate
E402   Potassium alginate
E403   Ammonium alginate
E404   Calcium alginate
E405   Propane-1,2-diol alginate (Propylene glycol alginate)
E407   Carrageenan
E410   Locust bean gum (Carob gum)
E413   Tragacanth
E414   Gum arabic (acacia)
 416   Karaya gum
 430   Polyoxyethylene (8) stearate
·431   Polyoxyethylene (40) stearate
 432   Polyoxyethylene (20) sorbitan monolaurate
 433   Polyoxyethylene (20) sorbitan mono-oleate
 434   Polyoxyethylene (20) sorbitan monopalmitate
 435   Polyoxyethylene (20) sorbitan monostearate
 436   Polyoxyethylene (20) sorbitan tristearate
E440(a) Pectin
E440(b) Amidated pectin
 442   Ammonium phosphatides
E460   { Microcrystalline cellulose
        { Alpha cellulose
E436   Hydroxypropylcellulose
E464   Hydroxypropylmethylcellulose
E465   Ethylmethylcellulose

E470	Sodium, potassium and calcium salts of fatty acids
E471	Mono- and di-glycerides of fatty acids
E472(a)	Acetic acid esters of mono- and di-glycerides of fatty acids
E472(b)	Lactic acid esters of mono- and di-glycerides of fatty acids
E472(c)	Citric acid esters of mono- and di-glycerides of fatty acids
E472(e)	Mono- and di-acetyltartaric acid esters of mono- and di-glycerides of fatty acids
E473	Sucrose esters of fatty acids
E474	Sucroglycerides
E475	Polyglycerol esters of polycondensed fatty acids of castor oil
E477	Propane-1,2-diol esters of fatty acids
478	Lactylated fatty acid esters of glycerol and propane-1,2-diol
E481	Sodium stearoyl-2-lactylate
E482	Calcium stearoyl-2-lactylate
E483	Stearyl tartrate
491	Sorbitan monostearate
492	Sorbitan tristearate
493	Sorbitan monolaurate
494	Sorbitan mono-oleate
495	Sorbitan monopalmitate
	Acetylated distarch glycerol
	Acetylated distarch phosphate
	Cholic acid
	Desoxycholic acid
	Dioctyl sodium sulphosuccinate
	Distarch glycerol
	Extract of quillaia
	Gelatine
	Hydroxypropyl distarch glycerol
	Hydroxypropyl starch
	Oxidatively polymerized soya bean oil
	Oxidized hydroxypropyl distarch glycerol
	Oxidized starch

Polyglycerol esters of dimerized fatty acids of soya
bean oil
Sorboyl palmitate
Stearyl citrate
Succinated mono-glycerides

Enzymes (no numbers)
Actinoplanes missouriensis — glucose isomerase
Aspergillus niger — glucose isomerase
Aspergillus oryzae var. — alpha-amylase and glucoamylase
Aspergillus oryzae — lipase
Aspergillus oryzae — protease
Bacillus coagulans — glucose isomerase
Bromelain
Carbohydrase, microbial, from *Aspergillus awamori*
Carbohydrase, microbial, from *Aspergillus niger*
Carbohydrase, microbial, from *Aspergillus oryzae*
Carbohydrase, microbial, from *Bacillus licheniformis*
Carbohydrase, microbial, from *Klebsiella aerogenes*
Carbohydrase, microbial, from *Rhizopus oryzae*
Carbohydrase, microbial, from *Saccharomyces*
Catalase
Catalase (bovine liver)
Catalase, microbial, from *Aspergillus niger*
Catalase, microbial, from *Micrococcus lisodeikticus*
Ficin
Lipase, animal
Malt carbohydrates
Mixed carbohydrates and protease, microbial, from *Bacillus subtilis*
Papain
Pepsin, avian
Pepsin (hog stomach)
Rennet
Rennet, bovine
Rennet, microbial, from *Bacillus cereus*
Rennet, microbial, from *Endothia parasitica*
Rennet, microbial, from *Mucor*
Streptomyces fradiae — protease

Streptomyces olivaceous — glucose isomerase
Streptomyces olivochromogenes — glucose isomerase
Streptomyces rubiginosus — glucose isomerase
Streptomyces violaceoniger — glucose isomerase
Trypsin

Firming Agents (E227–578)

E227	Calcium hydrogen sulphite
E333	Calcium citrate
E341(a)	*mono*Calcium phosphate, monobasic
516	Calcium sulphate
526	Calcium hydroxide
578	Calcium gluconate
	Aluminium ammonium sulphate
	Aluminium potassium sulphate
	Aluminium sodium sulphate
	Aluminium sulphate (anhydrous)
	Magnesium chloride
	Magnesium gluconate

Flavour Enhancers (620–637)

620	L-Glutamic acid
621	*mono*Sodium glutamate
622	*mono*Potassium glutamate
623	Calcium glutamate
627	Sodium guanylate
631	Sodium 5'-inosinate
635	Sodium 5'-ribonucleotide
636	Maltol
637	Ethyl maltol
	Ammonium glutamate
	Calcium 5'-guanylate
	Calcium 5'-inosinate
	Calcium 5'-ribonucleotide
	Guanylic acid
	Inosinic acid
	Magnesium glutamate
	Thaumatin

Flour Treatment Agents (E483–926)

E483	Stearyl tartrate
924	Potassium bromate
925	Chlorine
926	Chlorine dioxide
	Acetone peroxides
	Ammonium persulphate
	Calcium iodate
	Calcium peroxide
	Potassium iodate
	Potassium persulphate

Foam Stabilizers (E405–900)

E405	Propylene glycol alginate
E465	Ethylmethycellulose
900	Dimethylpolysiloxane
	Oxystearin
	Quillaia extracts

Gelling Agents (E400–508)

E400	Alginic acid
E401	Sodium alginate
E402	Potassium alginate
E404	Calcium alginate
E406	Agar
E407	Carrageenan
E410	Locust bean gum
E440(a)	Pectin
E440(b)	Amidated pectin
E450(a)	*tetra*Sodium diphosphate
E466	Carboxymethylcellulose, sodium salt
508	Potassium chloride
	Furcelleran (from *F. fastigiata*)
	Gelatin, edible

Glazing Agents (901–4)

901	Beeswax, white or yellow
903	Carnauba wax

904   Shellac

Humectants (350–E422)

350   Sodium hydrogen malate
E420(i)   Sorbitol
E420(ii)   Sorbitol syrup
E421   Mannitol
E422   Glycerol
           Polydextroses A and N
           Sodium lactate (solution)
           Triacetin
           Xylitol

Modified Starches (no numbers)

Acid-treated starch
Alkaline-treated starch
Bleached starch
Oxidized starches
Monostarch phosphate
Distarch glycerol
Distarch phosphate A esterified with sodium
    trimetaphosphate
Distarch phosphate B esterified with
    phosphorusoxychloride
Acetylated distarch phosphate
Acetylated distarch adipate
Acetylated distarch glycerol
Hydroxypropyl starch
Hydroxypropyl distarch glycerol
Hydroxypropyl distarch phosphate
Phosphated distarch phosphate

Preservatives (E200–E283)

E200   Sorbic acid
E201   Sodium sorbate
E202   Potassium sorbate
E203   Calcium sorbate
E210   Benzoic acid

E211   Sodium benzoate
E212   Potassium benzoate
E213   Calcium benzoate
E214   Ethyl 4-hydroxybenzoate (Ethyl para-hydroxybenzoate)
E215   Ethyl 4-hydroxybenzoate, sodium salt
E216   Propyl 4-hydroxybenzoate
E217   Propyl 4-hydroxybenzoate, sodium salt (sodium propyl para-hydroxybenzoate)
E218   Methyl 4-hydroxybenzoate (Methyl para-hydroxybenzoate)
E219   Methyl 4-hydroxybenzoate, sodium salt (Sodium methyl para-hydroxybenzoate)
E220   Sulphur dioxide
E221   Sodium sulphite
E222   Sodium hydrogen sulphite (Sodium bisulphite)
E223   Sodium metabisulphite
E226   Calcium sulphite
E227   Calcium hydrogen sulphite (Calcium bisulphite)
E230   Biphenyl (Diphenyl)
E231   2-Hydroxybiphenyl (Orthophenylphenol)
E232   Sodium biphenyl-2-yl oxide (Sodium orthophenylphenylate)
E233   2-(thiazol-4-yl) Benzimidazole (Thiabendazole)
234   Nisin
E239   Hexamine (Hexamethylenetetramine)
E249   Potassium nitrite
E250   Sodium nitrite
E251   Sodium nitrate
E252   Potassium nitrate
E280   Propionic acid
E281   Sodium propionate
E282   Calcium propionate
E283   Potassium propionate

Raising Agents (E341(a)–575)

E341(a)   *mono*Calcium phosphate monobasic
500   Sodium hydrogen carbonate

503	Ammonium carbonate
503	Ammonium hydrogen carbonate
541	Sodium aluminium phosphate, acidic
575	Glucono delta-lactone
	Ammonium phosphate, dibasic
	*mono*Ammonium orthophosphate

Sequestrants (E262–576)

E262	Sodium hydrogen diacetate
E330	Citric acid
E331	Sodium dihydrogen citrate
E331	*tri*Sodium citrate
E332	Potassium dihydrogen citrate
E332	*tri*Potassium citrate
E333	Calcium citrate
E334	Tartaric acid
E335	Sodium L-(+)-tartrate
E337	Potassium sodium L-(+)-tartrate
E339	*mono*Sodium monophosphate
E340(a)	*mono*Potassium monophosphate
E340(b)	*di*Potassium hydrogen orthophosphate
E340(c)	Potassium phosphate
385	Calcium disodium EDTA
E420(i)	Sorbitol
E420(ii)	Sorbitol syrup
E450(a)	*di*Sodium diphosphate
E450(a)	*di*Sodium pyrophosphate
E450(a)	*tri*Sodium phosphate
E450(a)	*tetra*Sodium diphosphate
E450(a)	*tetra*Potassium diphosphate
E450(c)	Sodium polyphosphates
E450(c)	Potassium polyphosphates
516	Calcium sulphate
544	Calcium polyphosphates
576	Sodium gluconate
	Citric and fatty acid esters of glycerol
	Isopropyl citrate mixture
	Oxystearin

Sodium triosulphate
Stearoyl citrate
Tartaric acid (DL)

Stabilizers (E331(c)–495)

E331(c)	*tri*Sodium citrate
E332	*tri*Potassium citrate
E335	Sodium L-(+)-tartrate
E337	Potassium sodium L-(+)-tartrate
E400	Alginic acid
E401	Sodium alginate
E402	Potassium alginate
E403	Ammonium alginate
E404	Calcium alginate
E405	Propane-1,2-diol alginate
E406	Agar
E407	Carrageenan
E410	Locust bean gum
E412	Guar gum
E413	Tragacanth
E414	Gum arabic
E415	Xanthan gum
416	Karaya gum
430	Polyoxyethylene (8) stearate
431	Polyoxyethylene (40) stearate
432	Polyoxyethylene (20) sorbitan monolaurate
433	Polyoxyethylene (20) sorbitan mono-oleate
434	Polyoxyethylene (20) sorbitan monopalmitate
435	Polyoxyethylene (20) sorbitan monostearate
436	Polyoxyethylene (20) sorbitan tristearate
E440(a)	Pectin
E440(b)	Amidated pectin
442	Ammonium phosphatides
E450(a)	*di*Sodium dihydrogen diphosphate
E460	Microcrystalline cellulose; alpha cellulose
E461	Methylcellulose
E463	Hydroxypropylcellulose
E464	Hydroxypropylmethylcellulose

E465	Ethylmethylcellulose
E466	Carboxymethylcellulose, sodium salt
E470	Sodium, potassium and calcium salts of fatty acids
E471	Mono- and di-glycerides of fatty acids
E472(a)	Acetic acid esters of mono- and di-glycerides of fatty acids
E472(b)	Lactic acid esters of mono- and di-glycerides of fatty acids
E472(c)	Citric acid esters of mono- and di-glycerides of fatty acids
E472(e)	Mono- and di-acetyltartaric acid esters of mono- and di-glycerides of fatty acids
E473	Sucrose esters of fatty acids
E474	Sucroglycerides
E475	Polyglycerol esters of fatty acids
476	Polyglycerol esters of polycondensed fatty acids of castor oil
E477	Propane-1,2-diol esters of fatty acids
478	Lactylated fatty acid esters of glycerol and propane-1,2-diol
E481	Sodium stearoyl-2-lactylate
E482	Calcium stearoyl-2-lactylate
E483	Stearoyl tartrate
491	Sorbitan monostearate
492	Sorbitan tristearate
493	Sorbitan monolaurate
494	Sorbitan mono-oleate
495	Sorbitan monopalmitate
	Acetylated distarch adipate
	Acid-treated starch
	Alkaline-treated starch
	Bleached starch
	Calcium acetate
	Dextrins, roasted starch, white and yellow
	Dioctyl sodium sulphosuccinate
	Distarch phosphate
	Extract of quillaia
	Furcelleran from *F. fastigiata*

Gelatin, edible
Gum ghatti
Modified starches
Monostarch phosphate
Oxidatively polymerized soya bean oil
Phosphated distarched phosphate
Polydextroses A and N
Polyglycerol esters dimerized fatty acids of soya
    bean oil
Polyvinylpyrrolidone
Sodium caseinate
Starch acetate esterified with acetic anhydride or
    vinyl acetate
Starch, sodium octenylsuccinate
Tara gum

Sweeteners (E420–E421)

E420	Sorbitol
E421	Mannitol
	Acesulfame potassium
	Aspartame
	Calcium saccharin
	Cyclohexylsulphamic acid
	Hydrogenated glucose syrup
	Isomaltitol
	Lactitol
	Saccharin
	Saccharin (potassium and sodium salts)
	Sodium cyclamate
	Sodium saccharin
	Thaumatin
	Xylitol

Thickeners (E400–E466)

E400	Alginic acid
E401	Sodium alginate
E402	Potassium alginate
E403	Ammonium alginate

E404	Calcium alginate
E405	Propane-1,2-diol alginate
E406	Agar
E407	Carageenan
E410	Locust bean gum
E412	Guar gum
E413	Tragacanth
E414	Gum arabic
E415	Xanthan gum
E416	Karaya gum
E440(a)	Pectin
E440(b)	Amidated pectin
E461	Methylcellulose
E463	Hydroxypropylcellulose
E464	Hydroxypropylmethylcellulose
E465	Ethylmethylcellulose
E466	Carboxymethylcellulose, sodium salt
	Acetylated distarch adipate
	Acetylated distarch glycerol
	Acetylated distarch phosphate
	Acid-treated starch
	Amylose and amylopectin
	Bleached starch
	Dextrins, roasted starch, white and yellow
	Distarch glycerol
	Distarch phosphate, A, esterified with sodium trimetaphosphate, B esterified with phosphorusoxychloride
	Furcelleran from *F. fastigiata*
	Gum ghatti
	Hydroxypropyl distarch glycerol
	Hydroxypropyl distarch phosphate
	Hydroxypropyl starch
	Modified starches
	Monostarch phosphate
	Oxidized hydroxypropyl distarch glycerol
	Oxidized starch
	Phosphated distarch phosphate

Polydextroses A and N
Starch acetate esterified with acetic anhydride or
   vinyl acetate
Starch, sodium octenylsuccinate
Starches, enzyme treated
Tara gum

Yeast Nutrients (E327–577)

E327	Calcium lactate
E332	Potassium dihydrogen citrate
E340(b)	*di*Potassium hydrogen orthophosphate
E341(b)	Calcium hydrogen orthophosphate
508	Potassium chloride
510	Ammonium chloride
516	Calcium sulphate
540	*di*Calcium pyrophosphate
576	Sodium gluconate
577	Potassium gluconate
	Ammonium phosphate, dibasic
	Calcium oxide
	Magnesium gluconate

Glossary of Additive Terms

Acid

Acids are added to foods either to impart a sour or sharp flavour or for technological reasons, to control the degree to which other substances in the food function. The acidity can thus be controlled in jams and preserves to provide the best level of setting that can be achieved by the fruit pectin. Substances which neutralize acids are called alkalis or bases; examples are sodium, calcium and ammonium hydroxide, and substances which can hold the acid-alkali balance at a constant level are known as buffers.

A.D.I.

The full acceptable daily intake (A.D.I.) for man, expressed on a body weight basis (mg/kg body weight) is the amount of food additive that can be taken daily in the diet, over a lifetime, without risk. It is allocated only to substances for which the available data include either the results of adequate short-term and long-term toxicological investigations or satisfactory information on the biochemistry and metabolic fate of the compound, or both.

The Joint WHO/FAO Expert Committee on Food Additives (JECFA) may allocate a full A.D.I. in cases where they are satisfied no further data are required, or a temporary A.D.I. in cases where some additional data are thought to be desirable. They must indicate to industry the time period within which the data must be submitted. If the data required are not submitted then the A.D.I. may be withdrawn. In practice, however, this rarely happens. There are currently no statutory A.D.I.'s in the UK except for preservatives.

Allergy

A reaction in which the body cannot effectively deal with a substance, usually a protein. We have an immune response to most foreign substances which enables our antibodies to remove them from the body by forming antigen/antibody complexes. Common foods which cause this kind of reaction are fish, eggs, shellfish, wheat, cow's milk and nuts, and recent work has shown that tartrazine (E102) increases plasma histamine levels in normal (non-sensitive) people as may certain other colours and preservatives.

Anti-caking Agents

These are substances which are added to foods such as icing sugar, salt or powdered milk to help them to flow freely and prevent the particles sticking together.

Anti-foaming Agents

These are substances added to food either to prevent excessive frothing on boiling, or to reduce the formation of scum, or to prevent boiling over. E900 Dimethylpolysiloxane, an inert silicone substance, is an example of an anti-foaming agent.

Antioxidants

Under normal circumstances, fats and oils slowly become oxidized when they are exposed to the oxygen in the atmosphere. The process is accompanied by the development of a rancid 'off' flavour and eating such food can cause sickness. The addition of antioxidants to the fats prevents the process of oxidation. Antioxidants are also added to other non-fat foods, such as cut fruits, to prevent discoloration brought about by oxidation. An example is lemon juice on cut apples when the natural antioxidants are Citric acid (E330) and Vitamin C (E300).

Artificial Sweeteners

These are substances, other than sugar, capable of producing a sweet taste.

Azo Dyes

An azo dye has a particular chemical structure of the atoms in its molecule. It could be this 'azo' construction within the molecule to which a proportion of the population is sensitive, or it might be impurities. About a fifth of people who are sensitive to aspirin (usually middle-aged adults and more commonly women than men) are also sensitive to azo dyes. Other groups which may be affected are asthmatics and people who suffer from eczema.

The kinds of reactions that occur in sensitive people are contractions of the bronchi — the tubes allowing air into the lungs — (and asthmatic attacks), nettle rash, watering eyes and nose, blurred vision, swelling of the skin with fluid, and in extreme cases shock and reduction in blood platelets with the production in the blood of anti-platelet antibodies. (The blood platelets are involved in blood clotting to seal wounds.)

It has been suggested by the late Dr Ben Feingold that azo dyes are among those substances which could trigger off the hyperactivity syndrome in children. The following are azo dyes:

E102	Tartrazine
E107	Yellow 2G
E110	Sunset yellow FCF
E122	Carmoisine
E123	Amaranth
E124	Ponceau 4R
E128	Red 2G
154	Brown FK
155	Chocolate brown HT
E151	Black PN
E180	Pigment rubine

'Coal tar dye' referes to dyes which were once made from coal tar but nowadays are made industrially. They may have the 'azo' configuration, or they may not. It includes all the above, plus:

E104	Quinoline yellow
E127	Erythrosine
E131	Patent blue V
E132	Indigo carmine
133	Brilliant blue FCF

Bases

Bases are added to foods to increase their alkalinity or reduce their acidity. Sometimes they are added to react with acids to give off carbon dioxide gas for aerating purposes.

BIBRA

British Industrial Biological Research Association.

Bleaching Agents

Substances employed to artificially bleach and whiten flour.

Buffers

Buffers are chemical substances which can resist considerable changes in the acid/alkali balance of solutions. The scale along which acid or alkali levels are measured is called the pH. Buffers (usually salts of weak acids) can maintain the pH at a predetermined level despite the addition of further acid or alkali.

Bulking Aids

Food additives which add to the bulk of the food but do not add to the calorific or energy value. The bulking aids are of value in slimming foods but they also help to 'pad out' or simulate more expensive ingredients.

Chelating Substances

When the acid/alkali ratio exceeds a particular limit or the ratio of traces of metal to one another exceeds a particular level, the trace metals may be precipitated out. The addition of a chelating substance such as EDTA (E385) retains the trace elements in the food solution, by bonding them on to an amino acid.

Coal Tar Dye

See azo dye. 'Coal tar' is *not* synonymous with 'azo' dye.

Colour Index (C.I.) Numbers

These colour reference numbers are allocated in the Colour Index of the Society of Dyers and Colourists (3rd Edition with 1975 revisions).

Colouring Matters

Water- or oil-soluble substances (or insoluble substances) which are produced artificially or are naturally occurring. Sometimes the colouring is permitted only on the outside of foods, especially confectionery, but usually it is permitted throughout the food.

COT

Committee on Toxicity of Chemicals in Food, Consumer Products and the Environment (DHSS)
The committee undertakes periodic reviews of existing permitted additives and approves new ones. Their advice and that of the FAC is presented to the Ministers of Health and Agriculture.

Diluents

Substances which are used to dilute other additives or to dissolve them.

Double-blind Trials

These are methods of testing drugs or additives without the subject knowing whether they are receiving the drug or not. If not, they would receive a placebo. The true effects of the drug can then be assessed.

Double-blind Crossover Trials

During the double-blind test (see above) the code-holder crosses over the drug and the placebo (page 354) without the knowledge of the experimenter or subject.

Emulsifiers

These are substances which can bring together oil, which is water-hating (hydrophobic) and water, which is lypophobic (fat-hating), and mix them so that they do not separate out into layers. Some emulsifiers are plant gums, some are chemicals and others are synthetically produced derivatives of natural products.

Emulsifying Salts

A mixture of salts such as citrates, phosphates and tartrates which is added to cheese when it is melted as part of its processing to prevent the 'stringiness' which normally occurs when cheese is cooked.

Enzymes
Natural protein catalysts which are responsible for most metabolic reactions in the living cell.

Excipients
This is the term for 'inactive' substances which are used to carry an 'active' drug in a tablet, capsule or elixir. The term is also applied in the baking industry to denote a carrier substance for additives used in bread.

FAC
Food Advisory Committee
Advises MAFF on the composition, labelling and advertising of food. It was formed in 1983 by the amalgamation of the Food Additives and Contaminants Committee and the Food Standards Committee.

Members do not sign the Official Secrets Act. MAFF has arranged that in future copies of toxicological data considered during reviews by the FAC will be available at the British Library. Regrettably, past data will not be available unless published.

Firming Agents
Calcium and magnesium salts are employed to retain the natural firmness or crispness of fruits and vegetables and to prevent their softening during the processing period.

Flavour Modifiers or Enhancers
These are substances used to enhance or reduce the taste or smell of a food without imparting any flavour of their own, so they are not 'flavours' as such, neither are they enzymes.

Food Intolerance
This is not to be confused with food allergy (see Allergy) which involves an immune response. It is also known as food idiosyncracy and pseudo-allergy.

One explanation is that the individual is deficient in the enzyme capable of metabolizing the food substance or ingredient. This may help to explain why young children may be more susceptible to some foods or ingredients: their metabolic activity is not developed. Substances such as *mono*Sodium glutamate (621) or caffeine provoke responses in intolerant people who lack the appropriate enzymes.

The symptoms may resemble those of food allergy when foods containing natural histamine, e.g. chocolate, strawberries, egg white, fish, or tomatoes, are consumed.

Gelling Agents

Substances which are capable of forming a jelly. Many of the gelling agents may be used in a stabilizing capacity too but not all stabilizers are capable of setting into a jelly.

Glazing Agents

Substances which either provide a shiny appearance or polish on the food, or provide a protective coat, or both.

Humectants

These are substances which absorb water vapour from the atmosphere and prevent the food from drying out and becoming hard and unpalatable. Glycerine is added to royal icing in the home as a humectant, to prevent the icing drying out and hardening.

JECFA

Joint Expert Committee on Food Additives
Composed of experts appointed by the Directors General of the World Health Organization (Geneva) and the Food and Agriculture Organization (Rome).

Liquid Freezants

Liquids or liquefiable gases which can freeze food by coming into contact with it directly and extracting heat from it.

Mineral Hydrocarbons

A wide variety of substances derived from bitumen (paraffin

hydrocarbons) whether liquid, semi-liquid or solid. The group includes white oil, liquid paraffin, petroleum jelly, microcrystalline wax and hard paraffin.

Mutation

A permanent change in the DNA-coded genetic material of the chromosomes, present in all body cells. When the cells divide, this change is passed on to subsequent generations of cells. This might have cancer-causing implications if it occurs in non-sexual cells, or reproductive implications (birth defects) if it happens in the ovaries or testes which produce the reproductive cells.

Packaging Gases

Inert gases, such as nitrogen, which are employed to occupy space in packaging which, if occupied by atmospheric air, would cause oxidation of the contents or encourage the growth of micro-organisms.

Placebo

An inactive substance or preparation given to satisfy the patient's symbolic need for drug therapy, and used in controlled studies to determine the efficacy of medicinal substances by giving some patients a placebo and some the medicine. Also, a procedure with no intrinsic therapeutic value performed for such a purpose.

Preservatives

Preservatives are substances which inhibit the growth of bacteria, fungi and viruses within foods and thus prevent the spoilage of these foods. Gases such as sulphur dioxide, organic and inorganic acids, phosphates and nitrates are all preservatives.

Propellants

Gases or volatile liquids employed in aerosol containers to expel the contents when the button is depressed.

Release Agents

Substances added to the machinery or coated on to food to prevent foods from sticking to the surfaces of food-processing equipment such as moulds, conveyors, cooking pans or trays. Release agents such as magnesium stearate are also added to tins in which foods are packaged to allow the contents to slip out easily.

SCF
Scientific Committee for Food
The committee and the working groups meet at the invitation of a representative of the European Economic Commission. The committee may be consulted by the Commission on any problem relating to the protection of the health and safety of persons arising from the consumption of food and in particular on the composition of food processes which are liable to modify food and the use of food additives and other processing aids, as well as the presence of contaminants.

Sequestrants
Traces of metals, always present in the environment, can cause deterioration in food by advancing the oxidation process, or cause premature setting in dessert mixes. Sequestrants are substances capable of attaching themselves to the trace metals such as calcium, iron or copper.

Solvents
These are liquids which are used to disperse substances either in solution or in suspension. They may also be used for extraction, then can either remain, as can be the case with the alcoholic extraction of a flavour, or be removed, as when oil is dissolved from seed.

Stabilizers
Similar in function to emulsifiers and thickeners, stabilizers serve to protect the droplets in an emulsion from collision with one another and consequently negate their tendency to separate out.

Stabilizers reduce coalescence either by adding to the viscosity or thickness of the medium forming a protection to the droplets or by forming protective colloids so that the frequency and energy of collisions are minimized. The term 'stabilizer' may embrace thickening and gelling agents.

Sweeteners

In the words of *The Sweeteners in Food Regulations 1983*, sweetener means 'any substance other than a carbohydrate, whose primary organoleptic (i.e. taste or 'mouth feel') characteristic is sweet.

There are twelve permitted sweeteners in Britain, three of which (mannitol, sorbitol and sorbitol syrup) already have E numbers (E421, E420). The others are:

Acesulfame potassium (Acesulfame K), a non-nutritive chemical, two hundred times as sweet as sugar.

Aspartame Prepared from two amino acids, phenylanyline and aspartic acid with about two hundred times the sweetness of sugar. It is safe except for people with phenylketonuria (PHK) because like many natural foods, *Aspartame* contains phenylanyline.

Hydrogenated glucose syrup (hydrogenated high maltose glucose) syrup prepared from glucose syrup.

Isomalt A complex molecule based on D-glucitol and D-mannitol.

Saccharin made from o-sulfamoylbenzoic acid.

Sodium saccharin sodium salt of o-sulfamoylbenzoic acid.

Calcium saccharin calcium salt of o-sulfamoylbenzoic acid.

(The name 'saccharin' includes the sodium and calcium salts.)

Thaumatin protein obtained by the aqueous extraction of the aries of the fruit of *Thaumatococcus daniellii*, a tropical plant found in Sierra Leone, Zaire, Sudan and Uganda. It has a licquorice after-taste.

Ice creams are not permitted to contain acesulfame potassium, aspartame, saccharin, sodium and calcium saccharin or thaumatin, but they are all permitted to be used in reduced sugar jam and similar products.

Synergists

A synergist is a substance which is capable of increasing or enhancing the effect of another substance. In the context of food additives, synergists are usually used to enhance the effects of antioxidants. These synergists include tartaric and citric acid and their calcium, potassium and sodium salts.

Tenderizer

A substance or process used to alter the structure of meat to make it less tough and more palatable. This is achieved by loosening the structure of the muscle fibres. There are three main types of tenderizing process:

(1) Mechanical, i.e. beating of meat to disrupt its structure.

(2) Ageing — as in the 'hanging' of game. Natural enzymes and micro-organisms start to decay the meat so loosening the structure.

(3) Artificial — proteins are broken down to their constituent amino acids in the gut by protein digesting (proteolytic) enzymes. Artificial tenderizers are concentrated forms of such enzymes used to disrupt the structure of meat. This is not a new idea. Four hundred years ago Cortez noted that Mexican Indians used to wrap tough meat in leaves from the papya tree. The leaves contain the protein digesting enzyme, papain. Another frequently used tenderizer is bromelain which comes from the pineapple.

Thickeners

Food additives which add to the viscosity of a food. Most of the thickeners employed are of plant origin; for example, seaweed or algae derivatives, or substances produced from cellulose capable of forming a gel or colloid. Silicon dioxide (551) is the only inorganic additive employed as a thickener.

Vitamins

Most vitamins are not regarded as food additives unless they are fulfilling the function of a food additive such as that of antioxidant in the case of E300 L-Ascorbic acid (vitamin C), E306–9 tocopherols (vitamin E), or a colour in the case of 101(a) riboflavin-5'-phosphate (vitamin B_2).

References

E102 Murdoch, R.D., Pollock, I., and Naeen, S., 'Tartrazine-induced Histamine Release in Vivo in Normal Subjects', paper presented at British Society for Allergy and Clinical Immunology Spring Meeting, 10 April 1987 (to be published October 1987).
— August, P.J., *Urticaria International Medicine Supplement* No. 6, 1983. Allergy 83: A symposium on recent developments in clinical allergy.
— Truswell, A. Stewart, 'ABC of Nutrition: Food Sensitivity', *British Medical Journal*, 1985, 951-5.
— Supramaniam, G. & Warner, J.O., 'Artificial Food Additive Intolerance in Patients with Angio-oedema and Urticaria', *The Lancet,* 18 October 1986.
— Hesser Lynn (BIBRA), 'Tartrazine on Trial', *Fd. Chem. Toxic.*, Vol. 22, No. 12, 1019-26, 1984. Quoting:

   Lockey, S., *An. Allergy*, 1959, 17, 719.
   Lockey, S., *An. Allergy*, 1977, 38, 206.
   Green, *An. Allergy*, 1974, 33, 274.
   Cordas, *J. Amer. Osteop. Assoc.*, 1978, 77, 696.
   Lahti, *Acta Derm-vener.*, 60, Suppl 91, Stockholm 1980.
   Warin & Smith, *Contact Dermatitis*, 1982, 8, 117.
   Trautlein & Mann, Ann, *Allergy*, 1978, 41, 28.
   Chafee & Settipane, J., *Allergy*, 1967, 40, 65.
   Criep, J., 'Allergy' *Clin. Immunology*, 1971, 48, 7.
   Settipane *et al, ibid*, 1976, 57, 541.
   Zlotlow & Settipane, *Amer. J. Clin. Nutr.*, 1977, 30, 1023.
   Mikkelsen *et al, Archives of Toxicology*, 1978, supplement 1, 141.
   Warin & Smith, *Br. J. Derm.*, 1976, 94, 401.
   Syvanen & Blackman, *Allergy*, Copenhagen, 1978, 33-342.
— Henschler, D. & Wild, D., 'Mutagenic Activity in Rat Urine after Feeding

with Azo Dye, tartrazine'. *Archives of Toxicology*, 57: 214–5, 1985.

— Egger, J., Carter, C.M., Graham, P.J., Gumley, D., Soothill, J.F., 'Controlled Trial of Oligoantigenic Treatment in the Hyperkinetic Syndrome', *The Lancet*, 9 March 1985.

E104 *Food Advisory Committee Final Report on the Review of the Colouring Matter in Food Regulations 1973*, MAFF, HMSO, 1987 quoting:
1) LEMM (1978), 'Metabolism and distribution studies in the rat and the dog of Quinoline Yellow or E104 labelled with 14C', unpublished report dated December 1978, Laboratoire d'Etudes du Métabolisme et Médicaments, Commissiariat à l'Energie Atomique, France (3 volumes and annexes), SUP 11501–5.

2) IFREB (1981), 'Carcinogenicity study of the OFI mouse with the colouring agent E104-Quinoline yellow', Report No. 110202 dated 2 October 1981, Institut Francais de Recherches et Essais Biologiques, St German-Sur-l'Arbrèsle, France, SUP 11501–11505.

3) Biodynamics Inc. (1973), 'A 3-generation reproduction study of D and C Yellow 10 in rats', unpublished Report No. 71R 740, dated 18 December 1973 submitted to the Cosmetic, Toiletry and Fragrance Association, Inc., by Biodynamics Inc., New Jersey, USA.

E110 Jacobson, M. F., Ph.D., *New England Journal of Medicine*, Vol. 313, #7, 15 August 1985, quoting 'Carcinogenic effect seen in preliminary report on FD and C yellow No. 6', *Food Chem. News.*, 1 October 1984, 19.

— Supramaniam, G. & Warner, J.O., 'Artificial Food Additive Intolerance in Patients with Angio-oedema and Urticaria', *The Lancet*, 18 October 1986.

E120 'Evaluation of Certain Food Additives', 25th Report of the Joint FAO/WHO Expert Committee on Food Additives, Technical Report Series 669, WHO, 1981, 19.

— Food Advisory Committee, 'Final Review of the Colouring Matter in Food Regulations 1973', FdAC/REP14, 1987.

E122 Traghi, E., Marinovich, M. & Galli, C.L., 'The Placental Transfer and Detection of ^{14}C-Carmoisine and Metabolites by HPLC Combined with a Radioactivity Monitor', *Disease Metabolism and Reproduction in the Toxic Response to Drugs and Other Chemicals, Archives of Toxicology*, Supplement 7, 312 (1984).

E123 Supramaniam, G. & Warner, J.O., 'Artificial Food Additive Intolerance in Patients with Angio-oedema and Urticaria', *The Lancet*, 18 October 1986.

— Taylor, R.J., *Food Additives*, John Wiley, 1980.

E127 Matula, T.I. & Downie, R.H., 'Genetic Toxicity of Erythrosine in yeast', *Mutation Research*, 138 (1984), 153–6.

— Jacobson, M. F., Ph.D., *New England Journal of Medicine*, Vol. 313 No. 7, 15 August 1985, quoting Molotsky, I., 'Heckler puts off action on barring use of six drugs', *New York Times*, 3 February 1985, 24.

— Colombi, M. & Wu, C.Y., 'A food dye, Erythrosine B, increases membrane permeability to calcium and other ions', *Biochem. Biophys. Acta*, 20 October 1981, 648(i) 49–54.

— Wenlock, R.W., Buss, D.H., Moxon, R.E., & Bunton, N.G., 'Trace Nutrients, 4 Iodine in British Food', *British Journal Nutrition* (1982), 47, 381–90.

— Katamine, Shinichiro et al, 'Differences in Bioavailability of Iodine among Iodine-rich Foods and Food Colours', *Nutrition Reports International*, Vol. 35 No.2, Feb. 87, and quoting Barbano, D.M. & Delaralle, M.E., 'Thermal degradation of FD and C Red No.3 and release of free iodide', *J. Food Prot.*, 47, 668–9 (1984).

128 WHO 1981 Technical Report, Series 669, 20.

— Combes, R.D. and Haveland-Smith, R.B., 'A Review of the Genotoxicity of Food, Drug and Cosmetic Colours and other Azo Triphenylmethane and Xanthene Dyes', *Mutation Research*, 93 (1982), 101–248.

E129 Combes, R.D. & Haveland-Smith, R.B., 'A Review of the Genotoxicity of Food, Drug and Cosmetic Colours and other Azo, Triphenylmethane and Xanthene Dyes', *Mutation Research*, 98 (1982), 112.

— 'Proposed an Additional Colour in the Commission Proposal for an 8th Amendment to the Colours Directive COM (85), 474 Final.'

— 'Annex 3 Report of the Scientific Committee for Food on Colouring Matters Authorized For Use in Foodstuffs Intended for Human Consumption.'

— MAFF 'Food Advisory Committee Final Review of the Colouring Matter in Food Regulations 1973', HMSO, 1987.

E132 Supramaniam, G. & Warner, J.O., 'Artificial Food Additive Intolerance in Patients with Angio-oedema and Urticaria', *The Lancet*, 18 October 1986.

— Jacobson, Michael F., *New England Journal of Medicine*, Vol.313 No.7, 15 August 1985.

— 'Food Advisory Committee Final Report of the Colouring Matter in Food Regulations 1973', HMSO, 1987.

E150 Wood, F., 'Caramel Colours under Review', *Nutrition Bulletin*, January 82, Vol.7 No.1.

— Spector, Reynold & Huntoon, Sheryl, 'Effects of Caramel Color (Ammonia Process) on Mammalian Vitamin B_6 Metabolism, *Toxicology and Applied Pharmacology*, 62, 172–8 (1982).

— Noltes, A.W. & Chappel, C.A., 'Toxicology of Caramel Colours: Current Status', *Food Toxicology — Real or Imaginary Problems*, ed. G.G. Gibson and R. Walker. Proceedings of an International Symposium at the University of Surrey, Guildford on 11–15 July 1983, Taylor and Francis, 1985.

154 Haveland-Smith, R.B. & Combes, R.D., Screening of food dyes for genotoxic activity, *Food and Cosmetic Toxicology*, 18, 1980, 215.

— Haveland-Smith, R.B. & Combes, R.D., 'Studies on the Genotoxicity of the Food Colour Brown FK and its Component Dyes using Bacterial Assays', *Mutation Research*, 105, 1982, 51.

— Venitt, S., and Bushell, C.T., 'Mutagenicity of the Food Colour Brown FK and Constituents in *Salmonella typhimurium*', *Mutation Research*, 40, 309.

— Combes, R.D., 'Brown FK and the colouring of smoked fish — a risk-benefit analysis, *Food Additives and Contaminants*, Vol.1 No.3, 1987.

E160(a) 'Carrots — do they combat cancer?' Citation of work under Prof. Nicholas Wald at St Bartholemew's Hospital in *Chemistry and Industry*, No.7, 205, 1 April 85.

E160(b) 'Evaluation of Certain Food Additives', Report of the Joint FAO/WHO Expert Committee on Food Additives Technical Report 683, Geneva 1982, 21.

E160(c) Personal communication with D.M. Taylor, T.C. Feeds Ltd, Gt Harwood, Blackburn, Lancs.

E160(g) Food Advisory Committee, 'Final Review of the Colouring Matter in Food Regulations 1973', FdAC/REP/4, HMSO 1987, 58–9.

E161(b&g) Personal communication with D.M. Taylor, T.C. Feeds Ltd, Gt Harwood, Blackburn, Lancs.

E163 'Evaluation of certain food additives', Report of the Joint FAO/WHO Expert Committee on Food Additives Technical Report, 683, Geneva 1982, 21.

E172 'Evaluation of Certain Food Additives', Technical Report Series 684 and 696, 23rd, 27th Report of the Joint FAO/WHO Expert Committee on Food Additives, WHO Geneva, 1980 and 1983.

E173 Bland, Jeffrey, *Your Personal Health Programme*, Thorsons, 1983, quoting D.P. Perl & C.J. Gibbs, 'Intraneuronal Aluminium Accumulation in Amyotrophic Lateral Sclerosis and Parkinsonism of Guam', *Science*, 217, 1053 (1982).

— Lerick, S.E., 'Dementia from Aluminium Pots', letter to *New England Journal of Medicine*, July 17 1980, 164.

— 'Aluminium dementia link', *Journal of Alternative Medicine*, June 85, quoting 'Acid rain may cause senile dementia', *New Scientist*, April 25 1985, & Lockie, A. 'Comparison of alumina — the drug picture', and 'Alzheimer's disease — the disease picture', *Brit. Hom. J.*, Vol. 73 2, 92–4 (1984), reviewed in *J.A.M.*'s March 1985 'Update'.

E200 Daniel, J.W., *Preservatives in Food Toxicology — Real or Imaginary Problems?* Proceedings of an International Symposium held at the University of Surrey, Guildford, on 11-15 July 1983, ed. G.G. Gibson and R. Walker, Taylor and Francis, 1985.

E210 August, P.J., 'Urticaria', *International Medicine Supplement*, 6 November 1983.

— Egger, J., Carter, C.M., Graham, P.J., Gumley, D., Soothill, J.F., 'Controlled Trial of Oligoantigenic Treatment in the Hyperkinetic Syndrome', *The Lancet*, 9 March 1985.

E211 Supramaniam, G. & Warner, J.O., 'Artificial Food Additive Intolerance in Patients with Angio-oedema and Urticaria', *The Lancet*, 18 October 1986.

E213 27th Report of the Joint FAO/WHO Expert Committee on Food Additives', Technical Report Series 696, Geneva 1983.

E214–216 Daniel, J.W., 'Preservatives' *in Food Toxicology — Real or Imaginary Problems?* Proceedings of an International Symposium held at the University of Surrey, Guildford, on 11-15 July 1983, ed. G.G. Gibson and R. Walker, Taylor and Francis, 1985.

E217–218 Tilmen, W.J. & Kuramoto, R., Martindale, 'The Extract Pharmacopoeia', quoting *Journal of the American Pharmaceutical Association, Scientific*, Vol.46 1957, 211.

E220 Weszicha, B., 'Sulphur dioxide in foods', *Nutrition Bulletin*, 42, Vol.9 (3), 155, 1984.

— Personal communication with Dr S.W. Brewer, University of Lancaster, Dept. of Chemistry.

— Yang, William H. & Purchase, Emerson C.R., 'Adverse Reactions to Sulfites', *Canadian Medical Association Journal*, Vol.133, 1 November 1985, p.865.

— Roger, L.J., Kehrl, H.R., Hazucha, M. & Horstman, 'Broncho Constriction in Asthmatics Exposed to Sulphur Dioxide during Repeated Exercise', *Journal of Applied Physiology* 59 (3): 784-791, 1985.

— Truswell, A. Stewart, 'ABC of Nutrition: Food Sensitivity', *British Medical Journal*, Vol.291, 5 October 1985, 951-5.

E221 Roger, L.J., Kehrl, H.R., Hazucha, M. & Horstman, 'Broncho Constriction in Asthmatics Exposed to Sulphur Dioxide during Repeated Exercise', *Journal of Applied Physiology* 59 (3): 784-791, 1985.

— Yang, William H. & Purchase, Emerson C.R., 'Adverse Reactions to Sulfites', *Canadian Medical Association Journal*, Vol. 133, 1 November 1985, 865.

— Personal communication with Dr S.W. Brewer, University of Lancaster, Dept. of Chemistry.

— Huang, A. *et al*, letter to *New England Journal of Medicine*, 23 August 1984, 542.

— *Medical World News*, 12 September 1983, 123.

— Levine, A.S., Labuza, T.P., Morley, J.E., letter in *New England Journal of Medicine*, 15 August 1985, 454.

E222 Roger, L.J., Kehrl, H.R., Hazucha, M. & Horstman, 'Broncho Constriction in Asthmatics Exposed to Sulphur Dioxide during Repeated Exercise', *Journal of Applied Physiology* 59 (3): 784-791, 1985.

— Personal communication with Dr S.W. Brewer, University of Lancaster, Dept. of Chemistry.

— Huang, A. *et al*, letter to *New England Journal of Medicine* 23 August 1984, 542.

— *Medical World News*, 12 September 1983, 123.

— Levine, A.S., Labuza, T.P., Morley, J.E., letter in *New England Journal of Medicine* 15 August 1985, 454.

— Yang, William H. & Purchase, Emerson C.R., 'Adverse reactions to Sulfites', *Canadian Medical Association Journal*, Vol. 133, 1 November 1985, 865.

E223 Supramaniam, G. & Warner, J.O., 'Artificial Food Additives Intolerance in Patients with Angio-oedema and Urticaria', *The Lancet*, 18 October 1986.

— Roger, L.J., Kehrl, H.R., Hazucha, M. & Horstman, 'Broncho Constriction in Asthmatics exposed to Sulphur Dioxide during Repeated Exercise', *Journal of Applied Physiology* 59 (3): 784-791, 1985.

— Yang, William H. & Purchase, Emerson C.R, 'Adverse reactions to Sulfites', *Canadian Medical Association Journal*, Vol. 133, 1 November 1985, 865.

— Levine, A.S., Labuza, T.P., Morley, J.E., letter in *New England Journal of Medicine*, 15 August 1985, 454.

— *Medical World News*, 12 September 1983, 123.

— Huang, A. *et al*, letter to *New England Journal of Medicine*, 23 August 1984, 542.

— Personal communication with Dr S.W. Brewer, University of Lancaster, Dept. of Chemistry.

— Truswell, A. Stewart, 'ABC of Nutrition: Food Sensitivity', *British Medical Journal*, Vol.291, 5 October 1985, 951-5.

E224 Roger, L.J., Kehrl, H.R., Hazucha, M. & Horstman, 'Broncho Constriction in Asthmatics Exposed to Sulphur Dioxide during Repeated Exercise', *Journal of Applied Physiology* 59 (3): 784-791, 1985.

— Jacobson, Michael F., *New England Journal of Medicine*, Vol. 313 No.7, 15 August 85.

E224–E227 Personal communication with Dr S.W. Brewer, University of Lancaster, Dept. of Chemistry.

— Huang A. *et al*, letter to *New England Journal of Medicine*, 23 August 1984, 542.

— *Medical World News*, 12 September 1983, 123.

— Yang, William H. & Purchase, Emerson C.R., 'Adverse reactions to sulfites', *Canadian Medical Association Journal*, Vol. 133, 1 November 1985, 865.

— Levine, A.S., Labuza, T.P., Morley, J.E., letter in *New England Journal of Medicine*, 15 August 1985, 454.

E249–E251 Weisburger, J.H., 'Role of Fat, Fiber, Nitrate and Food Additives in Carcinogens: a Critical Evaluation and Recommendation', *Nutrition and Cancer*, Vol.8, No.1, 1986.

E250 Tanaka, N., Meske, L., Doyle, M. & Traisman, E.A., '*Clostridium botulinum* challenge study on bacon made by the Wisconsin process — a three plant study', United States Department of Agriculture, 1984, quoted by Jacobson, M.F., in *The New England Journal of Medicine*, 15 August 1985.

E300–E321 Haigh, R., 'Safety and Necessity of Antioxidants: EEC Approach', *Food and Chemical Toxicology*, Vol.24 No.10/11, 1986, 1031-4.

E300 *New Scientist*, 16 January 1986.

E301 Kroes, R. & Wester, P.W., 'Forestomach Carcinogens: Possible Mechanisms of Action', *Food and Chemical Toxicology*, Vol. 24, No. 10/11, 1986 1085, quoting:

Mirrish, S.S., Pelfrene, A.F., Garcia, H. & Shubik, P., 'Effect of Sodium Ascorbate on Tumour Induction in Rats Treated With Morpholine and Sodium Nitrite and with Nitrosomorpholine', *Cancer Letters* (2), 101, 1976, and Fukishima, S. & Ito, N. (1985), 'Squamous Cell Carcinoma Forestomach Rat', in *Monographs on Pathology of Laboratory Animals' Digestive System*, ed. T.C. Jones, U. Mohr and R.D. Hunt, 292, Springer-Verlag, Berlin.

— Ito, N., Fukushima, S., Tsuda, H., Shirai, T., Hagiwara, A. & Imaida, K., 'Antioxidants: Carcinogenicity and Modifying Activity in Carcinogenesis', in *Toxicology — Real or Imaginary Problems?* Proceedings of an International Symposium held at the University of Guildford, Surrey, on 11-15 July 1983, ed. G.G. Gibson and R. Walker,

Taylor and Francis, 1985; quoting: Fukushima, S., Imaida, K., Sakata, T., Okamura, T., Shibata, M. & Ito, N., 1983, 'Promoting Effects of Sodium L-ascorbate on Two-stage Urinary Bladder Carcinogenesis in Rats', *Cancer Research*, 43, 4454-7.

E302 'Evaluation of Certain Food Additives', 25th Report of Joint FAO/WHO Expert Committee on Food Additives, TRS 669, 1981, WHO Geneva.

E304 Kahl, R. & Heildebrandt, A.G., 'Methodology for Studying Antioxidant Activity and Mechanisms of Action of Antioxidants', *Food and Chemical Toxicology*, Vol. 24 No. 10/11, 1007-14, 1986.

E306–E308 Lindsey, Jennifer A., Zhang, Hanfang, Kaasiki, Hisayuki, Morisaki, Nobuhiro, Sato, Takasi and Cornwell, 'Fatty Acid Metabolism and Cell Proliferation'; 'VII Antioxidant Effects of Tocopherols and Their Quinones', *Lipids*, Vol.20 No.3 (1985).

— Thomassi, G. and Silano, V., 'Assessment of the Safety of Tocopherols as Food Additives', *Food and Chemical Toxicology*, Vol. 24, No. 10/11, 1051-61, 1986.

E310 Kahl, R. and Heildebrandt, A.G., 'Methodology for Studying Antioxidant Activity and Mechanisms of Action of Antioxidants', *Food and Chemical Toxicology*, Vol. 24 No. 10/11, 1007-14, 1986.

E310–E312 Furia, *Handbook of Food Additives*, CRC, 1980.

E320 Furia, *Handbook of Food Additives*, CRC, 1980.

— Altmann, H.J., Wester, P.W., Matthiaschk, G., Grunow, W. & Van der Heijden, C.A., 'Induction of Early Lesions in the Forestomach of Rats by 3-tert-Butyl-4-hydroxyanisole (BHA). *Food and Chemical Toxicology*, Vol. 23, No. 8, 723-31, 1985.

— Altmann, H.J., Grunow, W., Mohr, U., Richter-Reichelm, H.B. & Wester, P.W., 'Effects of BHA and Related Phenols on the Forestomach of Rats', *Food and Chemical Toxicology*, Vol. 24, No. 10/11, 1183-8, 1986.

— Branen, A.L., Richardson, T., Goel, M.C., and Allen, J.R., 'Lipid and Enzyme Changes in the Blood and Liver of Monkeys Given Butylated Hydroxylene and Butylated Hydroxyanisole', *Food and Cosmetic Toxicology*, Vol. 11, 797-806, 1973.

— Cohen, L.A., Tanaka, T., Choi, K. & Weisburger, J.H., 'Paradoxical Behaviour of Dietary Butylated Hydroxianisole (BHA): Inhibition of Dimethylbenz(A)anthracene (DMBA)-induced Rat Mammary Tumors and Adrenal Nodules; Enhancement of Forestomach Lesions', photocopy of abstract.

— Conacher, A.S.B., Iverson, F., Lau, P.Y. & Page, B.D., 'Levels of BHA and BHT in Human and Animal Adipose Tissue: Interspecies Extrapolation', *Food and Chemical Toxicology*, Vol. 24, No. 10/11,

1159–62, 1986.

— Fisherman, E.W., Rossett, D., and Cohen, G. 'Serum Triglyceride and Cholesterol Levels and Lipid Electrophoretic Patterns in Intrinsic and Extrinsic Allergic States', *Annals of Allergy*, Vol. 38, January 1977.

— Ito, N., Fukushima, S., Tsuda, H., Shirai, T., Hagiwara, A., & Imaida, K., 'Antioxidants: Carcinogenicity and Modifying Activity in Tumorigenesis', in *Food Toxicology — Real or Imaginary Problems?* Proceedings of an International Symposium held at the University of Surrey, Guildford, on 11–15 July, 1983, ed. G.G. Gibson & R. Walker, Taylor and Francis.

— Ito, N., Fukushima, S., Shirai, T., Hagiwara, A., And Imaida, K., 'Drugs, Food Additives and Natural Products as Promoters in Rat Urinary Bladder Carcinogenesis', IART Scientific Publications 1984, Vol. 56 — *Models, Mechanisms and Etiology of Tumour Promoters*, 399–407.

— Kirkpatrick, D.C. & Lauer, B.H., 'Intake of Phenolic Antioxidants from Foods in Canada', *Food and Chemical Toxicology*, Vol. 24, No. 11/12, 1035–7, 1986.

— Kroes, R. & Wester, P.W., 'Forestomach Carcinogens: possible Mechanisms of Action', *Food and Chemical Toxicology*, Vol. 24, No. 10/11, 1083–9, 1986.

— Moch, R.W., 'Pathology of BHA- and BHT-induced Lesions', *Food and Chemical Toxicology*, Vol. 24, No. 10/11, 1167–9, 1986.

— Monroe, D.H., Holeski, C.J. & Eaton, D.L., 'Effects of Single-dose and Repeated-dose Pretreatment with 2(3)-tert-Butyl-4-hydroxyanisole (BHA) on the Hepatobiliary Disposition and Covalent Binding to DNA of Aflatoxin B_1 in the Rat', *Food and Chemical Toxicology*, Vol. 24, No. 12, 1273–81, 1986.

— Report of the Working Group on the Toxicology and Metabolism of Antioxidants, Dr W.G. Flamm (Chairman).

— Shamberger, R.J., 'Antioxidants and Cancer', in *Carcinogens and Mutagens in the Environment*, ed. Hans F. Stich, CRC Press Inc., Florida, 1982.

— Surak, J.G., Bradley, R.L., Branen, A.L., Maurer, A.J. & Ribelin, W.E., 'Butylated Hydroxyanisole (BHA) and Butylated Hydroxytoluene (BHT) Effects on Serum and Liver Lipid Levels in *Gallus domesticus*', *Poultry Science*, 56, 747–53, 1977.

— Talyor, M.J., Sharma, R.P. & Bourcier, D.R., 'Tissue Distribution and Pharmacokinetics of 3H-Butylated Hydroxyanisole in Female Mice', *Agents and Actions*, Vol. 15, 3/4 (1984).

— Tobe, M., Furuya, T., Kawasaki, Y., Naito, K., Sekita, K., Matsumoto, K., Ochiai, T., Usui, A., Kokubo, T., Kanno, J. and Hayashi, Y., 'Six-month

Toxicity Study of Butylated Hydroxyanisole in Beagle Dogs', *Food and Chemical Toxicology*, Vol. 24, No. 10/11, 1223-8, 1986.

— Wattenburg, L.W., 'Protective Effects of 2(3)-tert-Butyl-4-Hydroxyanisole on Chemical Carcinogenesis', *Food and Chemical Toxicology*, Vol. 24, No. 10/11, 1099-102, 1986.

— Wurtzen, G. & Olsen, P., 'BHA study in Pigs', *Food and Chemical Toxicology*, Vol. 24, No. 10/11, 1229-33, 1986.

E321 Furia, *Handbook of Food Additives*, CRC, 1980.

— Olsen, P. *et al*, *Pharmacologia et Toxicologia* 53(5), 433, 1983.

—Shamberger, R.J., 'Antioxidants and Cancer', Chapter 5 of *Carcinogens and Mutagens in the Environment*, ed. Hans F. Stich, Vol. II, 'Naturally Occurring Compounds, Endogenous Formation and Modulation', CRC Press Inc., Florida, 1982.

— Babich, H., 'Butylated Hydroxytoluene (BHT): A Review', *Environmental Research*, 29, 1–29 (1982).

— Fukayama, M.Y. & Hsieh, D.P.H., 'Effect of Butylated Hydroxytoluene Pretreatment on the Excretion, Tissue, Distribution and DNA Binding of (^{14}C) Aflatoxin B$_1$ in the Rat', *Food and Chemical Toxicology*, Vol. 23 No.6, 567-73.

— Branen, A.L., Richardson, T., Goel, M.C. & Allen, J.R., 'Lipid and Enzyme Changes in the Blood and Liver of Monkeys Given Butylated Hydroxylene and Butylated Hydroxanisole', *Food and Cosmetic Toxicology*, Vol. II, pp. 797-806, 1973.

— Brugh, M., 'Butylated Hydroxytoluene Protects Chickens Exposed to Newcastle Disease Virus', Department of Agriculture, Athens, Georgia, May 1977.

— Cohen, L.A., Choi, K., Numoto, S., Reddy, M., Berke, B. & Weisburger, J.H., 'Inhibition of Chemically Induced Mammary Carcinogenesis in Rats by Long-Term Exposure to Butylated Hydroxytoluene (BHT): Interrelations Among BHT Concentration, Carcinogen Dose and Diet', INCL Vol. 76, No. 4, April 1986.

— Conacher, A.S.B., Iverson, F., Lau, P.Y. & Page, B.D., 'Levels of BHA and BHT in Human and Animal Adipose Tissue: Interspecies Extrapolation', *Food and Chemical Toxicology*, Vol. 24, No. 10/11, 1159-62, 1986.

— Fisher, J.A., 'BHT as a Treatment for Herpes', *AntiAging News*, Vol. 3, No. 11, November 1983.

— Fisherman, E.W., Rossett, D. & Cohen, G., 'Serum Triglyceride and Cholesterol Levels and Lipid Electrophoretic Patterns in Intrinsic and Extrinsic Allergic States', *Annals of Allergy*, Vol. 38, January 1977.

— Haigh, R., 'Safety and Necessity of Antioxidants: EEC Approach', *Food and Chemical Toxicology*, Vol. 24, No. 10/11, 1031–4, 1986.

— Ito, N., Fukushima, S., Tsuda, H., Shirai, T., Hagiwara, A. & Imaida, K., 'Antioxidants: Carcinogenicity and Modifying Activity in Tumorigenesis', in *Food Toxicology — Real or Imaginary Problems?*, Proceedings of an International Symposium held at the University of Surrey, Guildford, on 11-15 July 1983, ed. G.G. Gibson and R. Walker, Taylor and Francis.

— Ito, N., Fukushima, S., Shirai, T., Hagiwara, A. & Imaida, K. 'Drugs, Food Additives and Natural Products as Promoters in Rat Urinary Bladder Carcinogenesis', IART Scientific Publications 1984, Vol. 56 — *Models, Mechanisms and Etiology of Tumour Promoters*, 399-407.

— Kirkpatrick, D.C. & Lauer, B.H., 'Intake of Phenolic Antioxidants from Foods in Canada', *Food and Chemical Toxicology*, Vol. 24, No. 11/12, 1035-7, 1986.

— Kroes, R. & Webster, P.W., 'Forestomach Carcinogens: Possible Mechanisms of Action', *Food and Chemical Toxicology*, Vol. 24, No. 10/11, 1083-89, 1986.

— Moch, R.W., 'Pathology of BHA and BHT-induced Lesions', *Food and Chemical Toxicology*, Vol. 24, No. 10/11, 1167-9, 1986.

— Moneret-Vautrin, D.A., Bene, M.C. & Faure, G., 'She Should Not Have Chewed', letter, *The Lancet*, 15 March 1986.

— Olsen, P., Bille, N. & Meyer, O., 'Hepatocellular Neoplasms in Rat Induced by Butylated Hydroxytoluene (BHT)', *Acta Pharmacol. et Toxicol.*, 1983, 53, 433-4.

— Olsen, P., Meyer, O., Bille, N. & Wurtzen, G., 'Carcinogenicity Study on Butylated Hydroxytoluene (BHT) in Winster Rats Exposed in Utero', *Food and Chemical Toxicology*, Vol. 24, No. 1, 1-12, 1986.

— Powell, C.J., Connelly, J.C., Jones, S.M., Grasso, P. & Bridges, J.W., 'Hepatic Responses to the Administration of High Doses of BHT to the Rat: Their Relevance to Hepatocarcinogenicity', *Food and Chemical Toxicology*, Vol. 24, No. 10/11, 1131-43, 1986.

— Report of the Working Group on the Toxicology and Metabolism of Antioxidants.

— Shamberger, R.J., 'Antioxidants and Cancer' in *Carcinogens and Mutagens in the Environment*, ed. Hans F. Stich, CRC Press Inc., Florida, 1982.

— Shilian, D.M. & Goldstone, J., 'Toxicity of Butylated Hydroxytoluene', letter to *The New England Journal of Medicine*, Vol. 314, No. 10, 6 March 1986, 648.

— Snipes, W., Person, S., Keith, A. & Cupp, J., 'Butylated Hydroxytoluene Inactivates Lipid-containing Viruses', *Science*, Vol. 118, 4 April 1975, 64-5.

— Surak, J.G., Bradley, R.L., Branen, A.L., Maurer, A.J. & Ribelin, W.E.,

'Butylated Hydroxyanisole (BHA) and Butylated Hydroxytoluene (BHT): Effects on Serum and Liver Lipid Levels in *Gallus domesticus*'. *Poultry Science*, 56, 747-53, 1977.

— Wursten, G. & Olsen, P. 'Chronic Study on BHT in Rats', *Food and Chemical Toxicology*, Vol. 24, No. 10/11, 1121-5, 1986.

E321(c) 'Process for giving flavour to broilers', *Food Processing Industry*, March 1982, i.

E338–341(a) Personal communications with L.R.J. Krakowicz, Albright & Wilson Ltd., Phosphates Division, PO Box 80, Trinity Street, Old Bury, Warley, West Midlands B69 4LN.

385 Haigh, R., 'Safety and Necessity of Antioxidants: EEC Approach', *Food and Chemical Toxicology*, 101, 24, No. 10/11, 1031-4, 1986.

E407 Abraham, R., Benitz, K.F., Mankes, R. & Rossenblum, I., 'Chronic and Subchronic Effects of Carrageenan in Rats', *Ecotoxicology and Environmental Safety*, 10, 173-83 (1985).

— Boxenbaum, H.G. & Dairman, W., 'Evaluation of an Animal Model for the Screening of Compounds Potentially Useful in Human Ulcerative Colitis: Effect of Salicylazosulfapyridine and Prednisolone on Carrageenan-induced Ulceration of the Large Intestine of the Guinea Pig', *Drug Development and Industrial Pharmacy*, 3 (2), 121-30 (1977).

— CECA SA (Satia) Food Applications — list of booklets and application data sheets, November 1984.

— Collins, T.F.X., Black, T.N. & Prew, J.H., 'Long-term Effects of Calcium Carrageenan in Rats — II, Effects on Foetal Development', *Food and Cosmetic Toxicology*, Vol. 15, 539-45, 1977.

— Engster, M. & Abraham, R. 'Cecal Response to Different Molecular Weights and Types of Carrageenan in the Guinea Pig', *Toxicology and Applied Pharmacology*, 38, 265-82 (1976).

— 'Evaluation of Certain Food Additives and Contaminants', 28th Report of the Joint FAO/WHO Expert Committee on Food Additives, Technical Report Series 710, WHO 1984.

— International Agency for Research on Cancer, *Monographs on the Evaluation of the Carcinogenic Risk of Chemicals to Man*, Lyons, France, Vol. 31, 1983.

— FMC, Marine Colloids Division, Box 308, Rockland Maine, 04841, 'Carrageenan, Current Regulatory Status for Safe Use in Food', personal communication, 16 August 1985.

— Personal communication with David W. Manning, Group Leader, Protein Section, Marine Colloids Division, FMC Corporation, 29 October 1985.

— Jensen, B.H., Andersen, J.O., Poulsen, S.S., Skrovolsen, S.,

Norbyrasmussen, Rasmussen S., Hansen, S.H., & Hvidberg, E.F., 'The Prophylactic Effect of 5-Amino-Salysilic Acid and Salazosulphapyridine on Degraded-Carrageenan-Induced Colitis in Guinea Pigs', *Scandinavian Journal of Gastroenterology*, 19 (1984).

— Mallett, A.K., Rowland, I.R., Bearne, Carol, A., & Nicklin, S., 'Influence of Dietary Carrageenans on Microbial Biotransformation Activities in the Cecum of Rodents and on Gastrointestinal Immune Status in the Rat', *Toxicology and Applied Pharmacology*, 78, 377-385 (1985).

— Marcus, R. & Watt, J., 'Seaweeds and Ulcerative Colitis in Laboratory Animals', letter to *The Lancet*, 30 August 1969, 489.

— Personal communication with Dr A.J. Marcus, 28 March 1985.

— Marcus, S.N., Marcus, A.J. & Watt, J., 'Chronic Ulcerative Disease of the Colon of Rabbits Fed Native Carrageenans', paper presented to the Proceedings of the Nutritional Society of Medicine, May 1983.

— Mottet, N.K., 'Carrageenan Ulceration as a Model for Human Ulcerative Colitis', letter to *The Lancet*, 26 December 1970.

— Thomson, A.W., Fowler, E.F., Sljivic, V.S. & Brent, L., 'Carrageenan Toxicity', letter to *The Lancet*, 10 May 1980.

— *Official Journal of the European Communities*, written answer by Lord Cockfield to written answer by Mr James Ford on the food additive carrageenan, 25 November 1985, No. C.304-9.

— Onderdonk, A.B., Franklin, M.L., & Cisneros, R.L., 'Production of Experiment Ulcerative Colitis in Gnotobiotic Guinea Pigs with Simplified Microflora', *Infection and Immunity*, April 1981, 225-31.

— Rustia, M., Shubik, P. & Patil, K., 'Lifespan Carcinogenicity Tests with Native Carrageenan in Rats and Hamsters', *Cancer Letters*, 11 (1980), 1-10.

— Watt, J., & Marcus, R., 'Harmful Effects of Carrageenan Fed to Animals', *Cancer Detection and Prevention*, 4 (1981), 129-34.

— Watt, J., Path, M.C. & Marcus, R., 'Hyperplastic Mucosal Changes in the Rabbit Colon Produced by Degraded Carrageenan', *Gastroenterology*, Vol. 59, No. 5, November 1970, 760-768.

— 'Toxicological Evaluation of Certain Food Additives and Contaminants' Joint FAO/WHO Expert Committee on Food Additives, Rome, 19-28 March 1984. WHO Food Additives series 1984, No. 19.

E412 Sharma, R.D., 'Hypocholesterolemic Activity of some Indian Gums', *Nutrition Research*, Vol. 4, 381-9, 1984.

— Tako, Masakuni & Nakamura, Sanehisa, 'Synergistic Interaction between Xanthan Gum and Guar Gum', *Carbohydrate Research*, 138 (1985), 207-13.

— Jenkins, D.J.A., Reynolds, D., Slarin, B., Leeds, A.R., Jenkins, A.L. & Jepson, E.M., 'Dietary fiber and blood lipids: treatment of hypercholesterolemia with guar crispbread', *The American Journal of Clinical Nutrition*, 33, March 1980, 575–81.

— McIvor, Michael E., Cummings, Charles C. & Mendeleff, Albert I., 'Long-term Ingestion of Guar Gum is not Toxic in Patients with Noninsulin Dependent Diabetes Mellitus', *The American Journal of Clinical Nutrition*, 41, May 1985, 891–4.

E413 Eastwood, M.A., Brydon, W.G. & Anderson, D.M.W., 'The Effects of Dietary Gum Tragacanth in Man', *Toxicology Letters*, 21, (1984), 73–81.

E414 Sharma, R.D., 'Hypocholesterolemic Activity of some Indian Gums', *Nutrition Research*, Vol. 4, 381–9, 1984.

— Anderson, D.M.W., 'Evidence for the safety of Guar Arabic (*Acacia senegal* (L) Willd.) as a Food Additive — a brief review', *Food Additives and Contaminants*, 1986, Vol. 3, No. 3, 225–30.

— McLean, A.H., Eastwood, M.A., Anderson, J.R. & Anderson, D.M.W., 'A Study on the Effects of Dietary Gum Arabic in Humans', *American Journal of Clinical Nutrition*, 37, March 1983, 368–75.

E415 Tako, Masakuni & Nakamura, Sanehisa, 'Synergistic Interaction between Xanthan Gum and Guar Gum', *Carbohydrate Research*, 138 (1985).

— Eastwood, M.A., Brydon, W.G. & Anderson, D.M.W., 'The Dietary Effects of Xanthan Gum in Man', *Food Additives and Contaminants* 1987, Vol. 4, No. 1, 17–26.

E416 Eastwood, M.A., Brydon, W.G. & Anderson, D.M.W., 'The Effects of Dietary Gum Karaya (*Sterculia*) in Man', *Toxicology Letters*, 17 (1983), 159–66.

E420 Review of the Soft Drinks Regulations 1964 (as amended), FSC/REP/65, MAFF, London, HMSO 1976.

E421(i) Conning, D.A., on the toxicity of diethylene glycol — written answer in *British Medical Journal*, Vol. 291, 2 November 1985.

E450(a,b & c) Personal communication with L.R.J. Krakowicz, Albright & Wilson Ltd., Phosphates Division, PO Box 80, Trinity Street, Old Bury, Warley, West Midlands B69 4LN.

E460 Mackler, Bradley, P. & Herbert, Victor, 'The Effect of Raw Wheat Bran, Alfalfa Meal and Alpha-cellulose on Iron Ascorbate Chelate and Ferric Chloride in three Binding Solutions', *The American Journal of Clinical Nutrition*, 42, October 1985, 618–28.

E461 Martindale, 'The Extract Pharmacopoeia', quoting Tilmen, W.J. & Karamoto, R., *Journal of the American Pharmaceutical Association, Scientific*, Vol. 46, 1957, 211.

E466 Anderson, D.M.W., Eastwood, M.A. & Brydon, W.G., 'The dietary effects of sodium carboxymethyl cellulose in man', *Food Hydrocolloids*,

Vol. 1, No. 1, 37-44, 1986.

E471 Hodge, D.G., 'Fat in Baked Products', *Nutrition Bulletin*, 48, Vol. 11 (3), 153, 1986, Flour Milling and Baking Research Association, Chorley Wood, Herts.

E474 Technical Report Series, 'Evaluation of Certain Food Additives', JECFA, WHO, Geneva, 1980.

476 Radiamuls 2253 'A flow improver for chocolate', Oleofina S.A., 37, rue de la Science, B-1040, Brussels.

500 Anonymous report, *New Scientist*, 5, 2 May 1985.

503 'Evaluation of certain food additives and contaminants', 26th Report of the Joint FAO/WHO Expert Committee on Food Additives, Technical Report Series 683, WHO 1982, 26.

509 'Food Additives in Focus', National Dairy Council, *Journal of Applied Physiology*, 59 (3), 784-91, 1985.

524 & 525 The Revised Codex Standard for Table Olives; personal communication with Miss B. Toole, Standards Division, Ministry of Agriculture, Fisheries and Food.

526 'Food Additives in Focus', National Dairy Council, *Journal of Applied Physiology*' 59 (3), 784-91, 1985.

540 & 541 Personal communication with L.R.J. Krakowicz, Albright & Wilson Ltd., Phosphates Division, PO Box 80, Trinity Street, Old Bury, Warley, West Midlands B69 4LN.

541 Lione, A., 'The Prophylactic Reduction of Aluminium Intake', *Food Chem. Toxical*, February 1983, 21 (1), 103-9.

— Katz, A.C., Frank, D.W., Sauerhoff, M.W., Zwicker, G.M., 'A Six-month Dietary Toxicity Study of Acidic Sodium Aluminium Phosphate in Beagle Dogs.' *Food and Chemical Toxicology*, January 1984 22(1), 7-9.

544 & 545 Personal communication with L.R.J. Krakowicz, Albright & Wilson Ltd., Phosphates Division, PO Box 80, Trinity Street, Old Bury, Warley, West Midlands B69 4LN.

554 & 556 Lione, A., 'The Prophylactic Reduction of Aluminium Intake, *Food Chemical Toxicol*, Vol. 21, No. 1, 103-9, 1983.

578 Kundu, P.N. & Das, A.A., 'Note on crossing experiments with *Aspergillus niger* for the production of calcium gluconate', *Journal of Applied Bacteriology*, 59, 1-5, 1985.

621 Truswell, A. Stewart, 'ABC of Nutrition Food Sensitivity', *British Medical Journal*, Vol. 291, 5 October 1985, 951-5.

— Noah, Norman D., 'Food Poisoning', *British Medical Journal*, Vol. 291, 28 September 1985, 879-83.

— Choi, Dennis, 'Glutamate Neurotoxicity in Cortical Cell Culture is Calcium Dependent', *Neuroscience Letters*, 58 (1985), 293-7.

— Olney, John W., Labruyere, Joan and de Gubareff, Taisija, 'Brain Damage in Mice From Voluntary Ingestion of Glutamate and Aspartate', *Neurobehavioural Toxicology*, Vol. 2, 125–9, 1980.

— Yamaguchi, Shizuko & Takahasi, Chikahito, 'Hedonic Functions of Monosodium Glutamate and Four Basic Taste Substances Used at Various Concentration Levels in Single and Complex Systems', *Agriculture and Biological Chemistry*, 48 (4), 1077–81, 1984.

— *Sweet, Sour, Salty, Bitter and Umami*, Umami Information Centre, Hosokawa Tsukiji Building, 1-9-9 Tsukiji, Chuo-ku, Tokyo 104, Japan.

— *What is MSG?*, Umami Information Centre, 5-8 Kyobashi 1-chome, Chuo-Ku, Tokyo 104, Japan.

— 'A Handbook for The World of Umami' (video), Umami Information Centre, 1986.

— *Proceedings of the International Symposium on MSG as Flavor Enhancer* (held on 8 December 1983 in Bangkok, Thailand), Ministry of Science, Technology and Energy, The Kingdom of Thailand.

— Kenny, R.A., 'The Chinese Restaurant Syndrome: An Anecdote Revisited', *Food and Chemical Toxicology*, Vol. 24, No. 4, 351–4, 1986.

— Yamaguchi, Shizuko & Takahasi, Chikahito, 'Interactions of Monosodium Glutamate and Sodium Chloride on Saltiness and Palatability of a Clear Soup', *Journal of Food Science*, Vol. 49, 1984.

— Stegink, L.D., Filer, L.J. Jnr. & Baker, G.L., 'Plasma Glutamate Concentrations in Adult Subjects Ingesting Monosodium L-glutamate in Consommé', *The American Journal of Clinical Nutrition*, 42, August 1985, 220–5.

— Wilkin, J.J. & Richmond, M.D., 'Does Monosodium Glutamate cause Flushing (or merely Glutamania)?', *Journal of the American Academy of Dermatology*, Vol. 15, No. 2, Part 1, August 1986.

621–3 Choi, Dennis, 'Glutamate Neurotoxicity in Cortical Cell Culture is Calcium Dependent', *Neuroscience Letters*, 58 (1985), 293–7.

907 IRAC monograph on the 'Evaluation of the Carcinogenic Risk of Chemicals to Man', Lyon, Vol. 3, 1973, 30.

— 'Recognized Carcinogens', IARC, 32; Dalton, A., Oil BSSRS, London, 1975, 47–8.

— Adrianova, M., *Voprosij Pitaniya*, Vol. 29, No. 5, 61, 1970: N1OSH (note QJ 6560000.

907 Lawrence, Felicity (ed.), *Additives, Your Complete Survival Guide*, Century, 1986.

920 Personal communication with Martin Dove, Croxton & Garry, Dorking.

924 Personal communication with J.E. Allen, British Bakeries, RHM

Centre, PO Box 178, Alma Road, Windsor, Berks SL4 3ST.
925 Taylor, R.J., *Food Additives*, John Wiley, 1980.

Bibliography

Bender, A.E., *Dictionary of Nutrition and Food Technology*, Butterworths Scientific Publications, 1960.

British Nutrition Foundation, *Why Additives? The Safety of Foods*, Forbes, 1987.

Brouk, B., *Plants Consumed by Man*, Academic Press, 1975.

Combes, R.D. & Haveland-Smith, R.B., 'A review of the genotoxicity of food, drug and cosmetic colours and other azo, triphenylmethane and xanthene dyes', *Mutation Research*, 98 (1982), 101-248.

Denner, W.H.B., 'Colourings and Preservatives in Food', *Human Nutrition: Applied Nutrition* (1984) 38A, 435-49 (E200, E201, E202, E203, E210, E211, E212, E213, E214, E215, E216, E217, E218, E219, E220, E221, E227, E230, E231, E232, E233, E239, E249, E250, E251, E252, E280, E281, E282, E283, E234).

Dorlands *Illustrated Medical Dictionary*, 26th Edition, W.B. Saunders.

FAO/WHO Food Additives Data System, FAO Food and Nutrition paper 30, based on the work of the Joint FAO/WHO Expert Committee on Food Additives, FAO, Rome, 1984.

Food Additives: The Balanced Approach, 1987. Free from MAFF, Freepost, Food Additives, Alnwick, Northumberland NE66 1BR.

Joint FAO/WHO Food Standards Programme, Codex Alimentarius Commission (1981), *Procedural Manual*, 5th edition. FAO/WHO, Rome.

HMSO, 1984 No 1305, 'The Food Labelling Regulations, 1984'.

HMSO, 'Report of the Review of Additives and Processing Aids used in the Production of Beer' (Food Additives and Contaminants Committee: FAC/REP/26, HMSO 1978).

Jacobson, Michael F., *Esters Digest. The Consumers' Factbook of Food Additives: Are they safe?* Anchor Books, Doubleday& Co. Inc., New York, 1976.

Jukes, D.J., *Food Legislation in the UK — a Concise Guide*, Butterworths, 1984.

Martindale, *The Extra Pharmacopoeia*, 28th Edition, 1982.

Miller, Melanie, 'Danger! Additives at Work', a Report on Food Additives, Their Use and Control, London Food Commission, October 1985.

Millstone, E., 'Food Additives: a technology out of control?' *New Scientist*, 18 October 1984.

Painter, A.A., *Meat Products and Spreadable Fish Products*, Special Report prepared for the Food and Drugs Industry. Bulletin December 84/January 1985 presented at a meeting of the Society of Chemical Industry Food Group.

National Dairy Council, *Food Additives in Focus*.

Pyke, M., *Food Science and Technology*, 4th edition 1981, John Murray.

Taylor, R.J., *Food Additives*, John Wiley, 1980.

Trease, G.E. & Evans, W.C., *Pharmacognosy*, 12th edn, Bailliere Tindall, 1983.

Walford, J., *Developments in Food Colours*, Elsevier, 1984.

Welham, R.D., 'The Early History of the Synthetic Dye Industry', *The Journal of the Society of Dyers and Colourists*, Vol. 79, Nos. 3, 4, & 5, 1963.

Windholz, Martha (editor), *The Merck Index 1976*, Merck and Co. Inc., Rathway, New Jersey.

Winter, R., *A Consumer's Dictionary of Food Additives*, Crown Publishers Inc., New York, 1984.

World Health Organization Evaluation of Certain Food Additives and Contaminants. Reports of the Joint FAO/WHO Expert Committee on Food Additives. Technical Report Series: 648 1980; 653 1980; 669 1981; 683 1982; 696 1983; Published by World Health Organization, Geneva.

Government Decrees

'Directive au conseil rélative au rapprochment des règlementations des Etats Membres concernant les matières colorantes pouvant être employées dans les denrées destinées à l'alimentation humaine', *Journal Officiel des Communautés Européennes*, Communauté Economique Européenne, 26 May 1962.

Council Directive of 25 July 1978 laying down specific criteria of purity for antioxidants which may be used in foodstuffs intended for human consumption, 77 & 78/664/EEC. *Official Journal of the European Communities*, 14 August 1978. Annexes to the above.

'Specific Criteria of Purity for Emulsifiers, Stabilizers, Thickeners and Gelling Agents for use in Food Stuffs', *Official Journal of the European Communities*, No. L 223/8, 14 August 1978.

Decree of the President of the Republic 26th March 1980 no. 327. 'Order implementing the law of 30th April 1962 no. 283 and subsequent amendments, governing hygiene standards in the production and sale of foodstuffs and beverages'. LTS 1561/82/Italian/BJH Circular No. 51.

Presidential Decree no. 322 of 18 May 1982, 'Implementation of EEC Directive No. 79/112 relating to the labelling of foodstuffs intended for sale to the ultimate consumer and the advertising of such foodstuffs, and the implementation of EEC Directive no. 77.94 on foodstuffs for particular nutritional use', LTS 574/82.

'Additives in Wine', *Oenological Practices For Wine*, Annex III to Regulations 337/79 published in *Official Journal of the European Communities* no. L54/34 of 5 March 1979; added by R.1990/80; amended by R.3577/81.

Italy (Food Legislation) 'Guide Prepared by Exporters to Europe', Branch Presidential Decree No. 337 of 26 March 1980 (*Gazzetta Ufficiale 193*, 16 July).

'Proposal for a Council Directive amending for the eighth time the Directive of 23 October 1962 on the Approximation of the rules of the Member States concerning the colouring matters authorized for use in foodstuffs intended for human consumption', Commission of the European Communities, COM (85) 474 final, Brussels, 19 September 1985.

Useful Addresses

Action Against Allergy
43 The Downs
London SW20 8HG
(will send detailed book list)

Allergy Laboratory
225 Putney Bridge Road,
London SW15 2PY
(cytotoxic tests and food antibody tests)

The Asthma Society
300 Upper Street
London N1 2XX
Tel: 01-226 2260

British Society for Allergy and Clinical Immunology
Paediatric Respiratory Unit
Cardiothoracic Institute
Brompton Hospital
Fulham Road
London SW3 6HP

Health Education Council
78 New Oxford Street
London WC1A 1AH

Hyperactive Children's Support Group
c/o Sally Bunday
71 Whyke Lane
Chichester
West Sussex PO19 2LD
Littlehampton (0903) 725182
(10am–3.30pm Monday–Friday)
(For information send SAE 9×4 inches)

Jigsaw (Allergic children)
Mrs B. Dickinson
7 Manor Road
Ducklington
Witney
(Postal group: please send SAE)

London Food Commission
88 Old Street
London EC1V 9AR
Tel: 01-253 9513

The Migraine Trust
45 Great Ormond Street
London WC1N 3HD
Tel: 01-278 2676

National Eczema Society
Tavistock House North
Tavistock Square
London WC1H 9SR
Tel: 01-388 4097

The Soil Association
86 Colston Street
Bristol
BS1 5BB
Tel: 0272 290661

Support for Parents of Allergic Children
Mrs J. Parkinson
31 Elm View
Streeton
W. Yorks
(SAE please)

Index

Ability and additives, 49–52
Absorption of chemicals, 299
Accuracy of labelling, 16–17, 18–19, 23, 25
Acid, 330, 347
Acidity regulators, 330
Activation, 297–9
Additive terms, 347–57
Additives
  alphabetical list and E numbers, 317–329
  avoidable, 57–60
  defined, 24
  disguise by, 25, 51–2, 57
  natural, 302
  nature-identical, 43, 302
  use of, 302
  see also: Labelling; Regulation of additives; Safety of additives; Testing
A.D.I. (acceptable daily intake), 27, 42, 303, 347–8
Advertising, accuracy of, 23, 61
  see also: Labelling
Alcoholic drinks, 27–31
Allergy, 41, 347–8, 378, 379, 380
Alternative test methods, 296–7, 299–300
Ames test, 299, 300
Anaemia, 78, 141
Angioedema, 70, 127
Animal tests, 296–7, 300, 301
Anti-caking agents, 331, 348
Anti-foaming agents, 331, 348
Antioxidants, 153–66, 331–2, 348
Argyria, 109
Aspirin-sensitivity, 55, 66, 69, 70, 73, 74, 75, 92, 114, 117, 118, 120, 160, 161, 162, 298, 349
Asthmatics, 27, 53, 55, 66, 69, 73, 75, 92, 106, 114, 116, 117, 118, 120, 124, 126–7, 127–8, 129, 130, 131, 160, 162, 378
Azo dyes, 348–9

Baby foods, 39, 55, 104, 138, 151, 160, 161, 162, 163, 166, 214, 216, 277, 281, 283, 284, 298
Bases, 350
Beer, 29–30
Behavioural problems and additives, 49–52, 303–4
BIBRA, 350
Bleaching agents, 350
Blood pressure problems, 80, 81
Bowel problems, 289
Brain dysfunction, 77
Bread and fresh foods, 32–3
Breathing problems, 80, 81
Buffers, 347, 350
Bulking aids, 350

Cagan, Dr Elizabeth, 49, 50, 51
Cancer, 59, 70, 74, 79, 90, 94, 138, 139, 140, 142, 163, 165, 203–4, 289, 291, 299, 300
  and pesticides, 45–6
Categories of additives, list of, 330–46
Cells, 297, 299, 300
Chelating substances, 350
Chemicals
  action of, 298–9
  use of, 294–5
  see also: Additives; Testing
Chicken, 35–6
Chinese Restaurant Syndrome, 277, 279
Chocolate and fancy confectionery, 31
Choice, freedom of, 23, 32, 37, 39, 61–2
Claims on labels, 18–20, 23
Coal tar dye, 349, 350

Colour Index numbers, 350
Colouring matters, 351
Colours, 30, 35-7, 38-42, 63-111, 302-3,
    332-4
    artificial, 40-2
    FAC Report, 30, 39, 42, 66, 295, 298
    functions of, 40
    natural, 42
    reduction of, 295, 298
    role of, 38-9
    and testing, 295
Confusion on labels, 23, 24
COT (Committee on Toxicity of
    Chemicals in Food), 309, 351
Curtis, Professor Frank, 42

Date marking, 17-18
Dermatitis, contact, 118, 119, 120, 208
Description of food (on label), 16
Detoxification, 297-8
Diabetics, 214
Diarrhoea, 87, 127, 153, 193, 208, 216,
    281, 291
Diluents, 351
Disguise by additives, 25, 51-2, 57
Diuretics, 135, 136
Dose, level of, 42
    and safety, 42
    and toxicity, 307

Eczema, 53, 349, 379
EEC Directive, 18
    and flavourings, 43-4
Eggs, 35-6, 37
Emulsifiers, Stabilizers and others,
    167-293, 334-6, 351
Emulsifying salts, 351-2
E Number Categories, 63-293
Environmental Protection Agency (EPA),
    45
Enzymes, 336-7, 352
Epidemiology, 295-6
Ethical considerations, 47-8
Excipients, 352

Fat content labelling, 26
Feingold, Dr Ben, 53, 54, 349
Feingold Diet, 50, 54
Firming agents, 337, 352
Flatulence, 200, 209, 214
Flavour modifiers, 352
Flavour enhancers, 337
Flavourings, 13, 43-4
Flour treatment agents, 338

Foam stabilizers, 338
Food Act, 43, 310-11
Food Advisory Committee (FAC), 30, 67,
    68-9, 70, 84, 97, 103, 105, 110, 111,
    295, 308, 352
    Report (1987), 30, 39, 42, 66, 295,
        298
Food enhancers, 352
Food Labelling Regulations, 19, **21-2,**
    27
    see also: Labelling
Food supplements, 23

Gastric upset, 70, 114, 127, 128, 131,
    137, 141, 160, 161, 162, 254
Gelling agents, 338, 353
Glazing agents, 338-9, 353
Goldenberg, Dr Nathan, 39
Gout, 282, 283, 284

Humectants, 339, 353
Hyperactive Children's Support Group,
    54, 66, 69, 70, 72, 73, 75, 78, 80, 89,
    92, 95, 115, 116, 117, 118, 119, 120,
    121, 124, 127, 129, 130, 131, 132, 138,
    139, 140, 166, 379
    see also: Hyperactivity
Hyperactivity, 50, 53-6, 66, 303-4, 349
    symptoms of, 349
    see also: Hyperactive Children's
        Support Group

Information
    accurate, 23
    inaccurate, 16-17, 305
    lack of, 31, 44
    see also: Labelling
Ingredient labelling, 13-17, 30-4
Ingredients
    additives in, 32
    secret, 27-34
Intolerance, food, 303-4, 352-3
Itching, 67, 80, 81

JECFA (Joint Expert Committee on Food
    Additives), 117, 155, 181, 230, 233,
    234, 267, 353

Kidney damage, 193
Kidney problems, 141, 216, 227, 228,
    229, 230, 233, 234

Labelling, 13-26, **14, 15,** 302, 309-12
    accuracy of, 16-17, 18-19, 23, 25, 61

contents clearly defined, 43
ingredient, 13–17, 30–4
and pesticides, 45
regulation, 19, **21–2,** 27
and religious groups, 47–8
unwrapped food, 32–3
voluntary, 26, 31, 33, 34
see also: Information
Labelling of Food Regulations, 19,
21–2, 27
see also: Labelling
Legislation, problems with, 18, 23, 33
see also: Regulations
Liquid freezants, 353
Loopholes in regulations, 32–3, 37, 44

Manufacturers
and accuracy of labelling, 16–17, 25,
31, 302
and claims, 23
and profit, 61–2
voluntary labelling, 26, 31, 33, 34
Meat products, 24–6
Medicines, 33–4
Mathemoglobinemia, 138, 139
Migraine, 66, 148, 149, 150, 379
Mineral hydrocarbons, 353–4
Minerals, 19–23, **22**
Misleading information, 16–17
Modified starches, 339
Mouth
numbing of, 118, 119, 120, 121, 122
ulcers, 174, 175
Mucous membranes, irritation of, 252,
292
Mutation, 354

Nausea, 80, 81, 127, 132, 216, 254, 281,
291
'Need', assessment of, 309, **310–11**
for additives, 40, 42, 51
Neurological disorders, 115
Non-kosher food additives, 47–8
Nitrosation, 298
Nutritional purpose foods, special, 18

Oedema, 73
Organically-grown foods, 46

Packaging gases, 354
Parkinson-type diseases, 108, 265, 266
Perkin, Sir William Henry, 41
Pesticides, 45–6
Phototoxicity, 77

Pigments, use of, 37
see also: Colours
Placebo, 354
Polyunsaturated fatty acids, 18–19
Prediction of toxicity, 296, 301
see also: Testing
Preservatives, 111–51, 339–40, 354
Propellants, 354

Raising agents, 340–1
Recommended Daily Amounts, 23
Regulations, 16, 24–5, 32–3, 295, 301
abuse of, 33
of additives, 308–16
list of, 312–16
FAC Report (1987), 30, 39, 42, 66,
295, 298
Food Labelling, 19, **21–2,** 27
loopholes in, 32–3, 37, 44
and secrecy, 308
see also: Legislation
Release agents, 354–5
Religious groups, needs of, 47–8
Retina, spotting of, 103
Rhinitis, 67

Safety of additives, 44, 302
assessment of, 294–304
proof of, 296–7
SCF (Scientific Committee for Food),
355
Schaus, Alexander G., 49–50, 52
Senile dementia, 108, 265, 266, 271,
272
Sequestrants, 341–2, 355
Shelf-life, 17
Short term assays, 299, 300–1
Skeletal abnormalities, 109, 134
Skin sensitivity, 67, 80, 92, 111, 121, 122,
128, 129, 130, 131, 132, 137, 160, 174,
219, 287
Soil Association, the, 46, 379
Solvents, 355
Stabilizers, 342–4, 355
Sweeteners, artificial, 344, 348, 356
Synergeists, 356

Teeth, erosion of, 153, 171
Tenderizer, 357
Testing, 294–304
alternative, 296–7
animal, 296–7, 300, 301
conclusions, 296
procedures, 295

tier system, 301
Thickeners, 344-6, 357
Thyroid problems, 77
Tier system of testing, 301
Tissue culture tests, 299
Toxicity of flavours, 43
Toxicity testing, 294-304
Trading Standards Officer, 17, 33
Trials
  double-blind, 351
  double-blind crossover, 66, 351
Trout and salmon, 36-7

Urine disorders, 135, 137, 193, 216, 218,
  252

Urticaria, 66, 70, 73, 74, 80, 92, 98, 114,
  116, 117, 118, 120, 127, 128, 137, 160,
  165, 218, 219, 287, 288

Villejuif List, the, 305-7, **306-7**
Vitamins, 19-23, **21,** 357
Vomiting, 70, 81, 132, 193, 216, 254,
  281, 291

Water, added, 13, 24-5, 32-3
Weight of ingredients, 13-16
Whitehead, Dr Roger, 23
Wine, 27-9, 48

Yeast nutrients, 346